Adventures In Chinese Medicine:

Acupuncture, Herbs, And Ancient Ideas
For Today

Jennifer Dubowsky, L.A.c.

Acknowledgments

I would like to thank the people who contributed their own experiences and knowledge to this book: Laurie ShoulterKarall (an extra thank you to Laurie for help with the editing), Kai Tao, Nicole Hohmann and Diane Lowry. I would also like to thank Christina Shaver and Jennifer Chertow for their enthusiasm, suggestions and support. Thank you to Azhar Ehasn for bringing my superhero vision to life. To my family, Dan, Shrim, Keira and Priya, as well as to my dear friends, thank you for your love and encouragement. Most of all, a huge thank you to my mother, Dr. Linda Edelstein, who was my editor, critic, inspiration and cheerleader. I couldn't have done it without you!

Table of contents

Intention

Welcome to the world of Traditional Chinese Medicine. This book is an invitation to join me on an adventure into ideas and practices that may be new to some of you, and will hopefully be intriguing to all of you. These pages offer an introduction to Traditional Chinese Medicine (TCM) and I will be your guide for the journey. Like any helpful guide in an unfamiliar place, I want to make your visit rewarding and friendly so that you will be comfortable, enjoy your stay, return often, and benefit from the enormous healing potential of the diverse techniques offered by TCM.

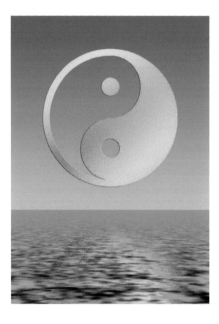

My intention in writing this book is to provide you with an easy to read, enjoyable overview of some of the best known concepts and commonly used modalities in TCM, such as acupuncture, Chinese herbal medicine and cupping. TCM is a vast topic with many important concepts and tools. I have chosen to touch on the ideas and techniques that you will find most useful and that are used regularly in offices throughout the United States and in many other countries. I want to share my passion for TCM with you by translating the basic, important elements of Traditional Chinese Medicine and explaining how these ancient techniques can change your life. I can't cover all of TCM and I won't try. As in any complex field, there is always more to understand.

Because Traditional Chinese Medicine originated in an ancient civilization, before there was a written language, the terms that are used to describe ailments, diagnosis, and treatments are often unrecognizable to people who do not have some training in the field, but that is exactly why you have a guide!

In the thousands of years that TCM has been developing in Asian countries, many scholars and practitioners have written about their theories, viewpoints and techniques. Gifted medical practitioners and philosophers, much wiser than I, have produced countless writings. Unfortunately, much of their work is hard to decipher and deters potential enthusiasts rather than inviting them to go further. In this book, you will find writing that you can understand, relate to, and hopefully find intriguing.

My desire is that more people comprehend and appreciate Chinese Medicine. It is a fascinating field, with concepts that changed how I view the world. It has a great deal to offer you, too. Traditional Chinese Medicine is more than medical techniques; it is the rooted in the philosophy of yin and yang which is all about balance. By finding balance in our lives and making conscious choices, we can greatly influence and improve the quality of our lives and the health of our bodies.

Who should read this book? If you are considering trying Chinese Medicine to help you feel better; if you are simply interested in this holistic approach to health; if you think you want to go to school for training in TCM; if you teach people who are beginning school in this field; and especially if you are a patient or treat patients who want to learn more about the practices and ideas that guide the methods, this book is for you. I have organized the book into chapters and included pictures, photos, diagrams and charts to make the information as user friendly as possible.

Definitions

There are many Chinese Medicine terms used in this book and some of them may be unfamiliar to you. Don't worry. Whenever I first use a term in a chapter, I define it. Also, to get you started, I'm defining many common terms, concepts, and techniques below. In this way, you can refer back to them and have an easy reference page of these complex ideas.

Acupuncture - A technique that involves the insertion of a very fine needle into a specific point on your body (usually on a meridian) in order to encourage balance and healing.

Acupoint - Another term for an acupuncture point.

Acupressure - The use of pressure on an acupoint instead of a needle to stimulate the point.

Chinese Herbal Medicine - Herbal remedies refer to the use of the healing properties of plants, flowers, minerals and animal sources. Herbs are available in many forms including, tablets, teas, and tinctures.

Cupping Therapy - Special cups are used to create suction on specific parts of your body. They draw out disease and toxins and can also be used to relieve pain and loosen muscles.

Meridians - Pathways of Qi that have been mapped out by Chinese Medicine practitioners over thousands of years. The majority of acupuncture points are found on meridians.

Moxabustion - Often called 'Moxa", this healing technique applies the heated herb mugwort near your skin to stimulate and warm acupuncture points.

Pattern Diagnosis - A system by which your practitioner determines and explains your symptoms.

Qi - A nonmaterial but fundamental, essential substance that is at the core of something as large as our universe and as personal as our own selves. Some people think of Qi as life energy. As energy, Qi travels along the meridians in your body and is manipulated by your acupuncturist in order to achieve better health for you.

Stagnation - A common TCM diagnostic term that refers to Qi or fluids that are not flowing freely or are unmoving.

The Five Elements - A Chinese Medicine concept that illustrates the relationship between our environment and ourselves by using 5 common elements: Fire; Water; Wood; Metal; and Earth.

Tui na - Tui na is a medicinal form of Chinese massage.

Yin and Yang - Essential concepts that demonstrate the constantly changing interactions in the universe. The ebb and flow of yin and yang, light and dark, activity and rest, creation and destruction, reminds us that everything is in motion and constantly influencing our lives and the nature in which we live.

Yang - Is the more masculine, hot, active, light and creative energy.

Yin - The opposite of yang. Yin is considered more feminine, cooler, nourishing and the energy of evening.

Chapter 1 - The Adventure Begins....

Traditional Chinese Medicine (TCM) is a natural, holistic healing system that has been in use for thousands of years. Using the knowledge that has been compiled and refined over centuries, Chinese Medicine works to restore harmony and energetic balance to your body, thereby stimulating natural healing and promoting health. TCM may sound mystical to you but it is widely used today in clinics and hospitals throughout China and in most areas of Asia as a primary medical modality. In the last 50 years, there has been a growing demand for TCM practices all over the world as people realize the benefits provided.

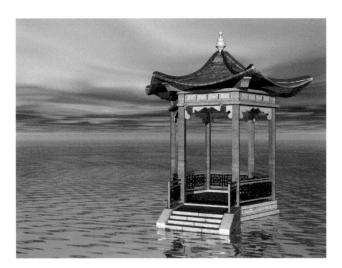

The techniques of TCM are designed to help your body regain, create, and maintain health. These days, most people who practice Traditional Chinese Medicine in the United States have achieved their knowledge by graduating from a four year Masters Program and then receiving a diplomate by passing a National exam given by the NCCAOM (National Certification Commission for Acupuncture and Oriental Medicine). After all that, most states have additional requirements to meet before you can practice.

Chinese Medicine is vast in its knowledge and methods of treating people. Some of the more commonly known techniques are Acupuncture, Cupping and Herbal Medicine. There are other tools and diagnostic procedures that may be unfamiliar to you now, but by the end of this book, you will have a better understanding and appreciation of Chinese Medicine.

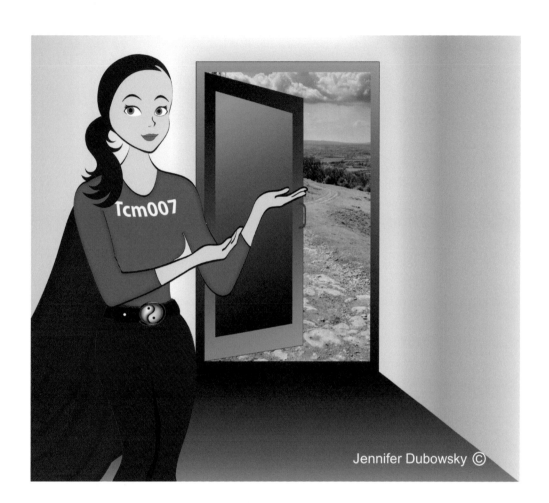

Chapter 2 - A Brief History Of Chinese Medicine

Ancient Beginnings

Chinese Medicine has been used for thousands of years and pre-dates recorded history so there are many versions of 'the beginning'. We have more information, scarce as it is, about the history of acupuncture than about other techniques. Some scholars date pre-acupuncture techniques to an ancient period, the Later Stone Age (prior to 6000 B.C.E.), before people had learned to cast iron but when they were able to sharpen stone into tools. One such implement, known as bian, was a stone that had been chiseled to a knife-like tip or edge. It was used for bloodletting and 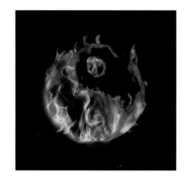 to lance abscesses and boils. One of these tools was found in Duolon County, Mongolia, in 1963, and is considered to be a likely precursor to modern acupuncture needles. In the Neolithic Period (6000 B.C.E. - 2000 B.C.E.), the use of tools became widespread. Still later, during the Han Dynasty (206 B.C.E. – 24 A.C.E.), as tools became increasingly sophisticated, stone and bone needles were replaced with metal medical implements, much closer to those we use today and a tremendous step forward.

Acupuncture is simply the best known technique in Chinese Medicine but TCM has always included a variety of creative healing methods. Cupping, the art of placing suction cups on specific areas of your body, was mentioned 3000 years ago. Moxabustion, the technique of burning a small piece of the herb mugwort close to the skin, is recorded in hieroglyphs and pictographs that date back to 1600 B.C.E. - 1100 B.C.E. The history of these unique Chinese Medicine treatments: Acupuncture, Cupping, Moxabustion, and others will be explained in their own chapters later in the book.

I offer these brief historical facts to remind you that, although Chinese Medicine is considered new and unusual in the United States, we are a comparatively young country, and these methods have been developed and practiced successfully in other countries for thousands of years.

As we move through the various practices of Chinese Medicine, you may be struck, as I was, by noticeable differences from the more familiar, conventional Western practices. One very important distinction between Eastern and Western medicine is that they come from very different philosophical roots. Western medicine depends heavily on science, with its ideological roots in Greece and Egypt. Rene Descartes (1596-1650), the famous French philosopher and one of the fathers of modern science and mathematics, greatly influenced the formation of the scientific method. As a scientist, in order to get bodies to dissect, he made a deal with the Pope that medicine would confine itself to the body. People's emotions and souls would be the province of the Church. This overly simplistic explanation points out the evolution of Western medicine's creation of a separation of mind and body, viewing the body as a complex system of biological parts, rather than a holistic unit. Certainly Western medicine has accomplished amazing things, but it is not the only path to wellness.

From a different origin, the philosophy that guides Chinese Medicine is rooted in the 8000 year old Taoist tradition. It focuses on a person's relationship with nature and the universe, reflecting the classical Chinese belief that, as human beings, we live in intimate connectedness with our environment. It is said that a legendary sage named Fu Hsu, living in the Yellow River area of China approximately 8000 years ago, came up with two symbols based on his observations of nature. He believed that these symbols, a broken line (representing yin) and an unbroken line (representing yang), illustrate the two major forces in the cosmos.

————— —————   ———————————
            yin   yang

From this idea, Fu Hsu formulated the well known concept of yin and yang, vital to Chinese Medicine theory and practice. This philosophy that began thousands of years ago in China with reflections on the universe and our place in the cosmos remains the basis of Chinese Medicine theory today.

2000 Years In 958 Words

You would need complete courses in Chinese history, philosophy and medicine to learn all of the major advancements that have taken

12

place in the field of Chinese Medicine in the last two thousand years. However, I do want to provide a timeline of the most notable achievements in TCM from 421 B.C.E. until today. The dates are approximate and depend on your source.

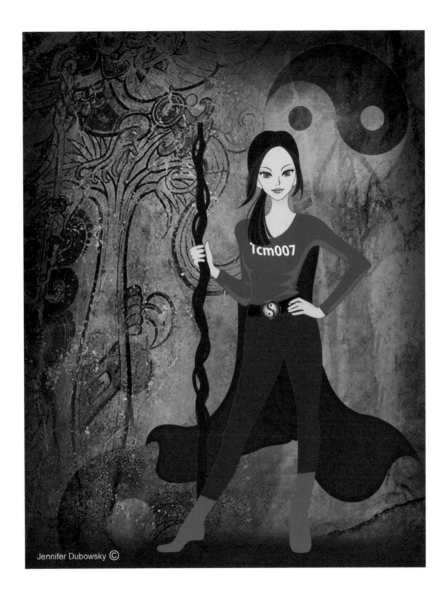

Jennifer Dubowsky ©

▶ **421 B.C.E. to 221 B.C.E.** - Chinese Medicine made great strides during the Warring States Era. The concepts that evolved during these years provide the foundation for today's practices and there was a convergence of Chinese thought and ideas about acupuncture that lasted until the Communist revolution of the 1940s. The most significant medical milestone of this time was the *The Yellow Emperor's Classic of Internal Medicine*, the *Nei Jing*. The *Nei Jing* is the oldest known

Chinese Medical text, possibly the oldest medical text. This famous text is considered 'the bible' of Chinese Medicine. It was compiled around 305-204 B.C. and consists of two parts:

The Su Wen - Plain Questions is the first part which covers, but is not limited to, anatomy and physiology, pathology, diagnosis, differentiation of syndromes, yin-yang, five elements, treatment, and our relationship with nature and the cosmos.

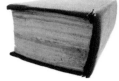

The Ling Shu - Miraculous Pivot/Spiritual Axis is the second part and focuses on acupuncture and moxabustion. Another well known text of this period is the *Nan Jing*, meaning *Book of Difficult Questions* which discusses the five element theory, hara diagnosis, eight extra meridians, and other important topics.

▶ **220 A.D. -** The *Shang Han Lun* is a classic book about Chinese herbal medicine that contains 200 formulas and was written by doctor Jiang Zhongjing.

▶ **1368 A.D. to 1644 A.D. -** During the Ming dynasty, the number of herbal formulas in the official pharmacopeias of Chinese medicine grew to 10,000. It was a rich time for Chinese Medicine because classic texts were revised and use of acupuncture advanced as treatments were refined and additional points outside the main meridians were added. Moxa sticks were developed to provide safe results using indirect heat treatments. In 1601, the encyclopedic work of 120 volumes called the *Principle and Practice of Medicine* was written by the famous physician Wang Gendung. That same year, Yang Jizhou wrote *Zhenjin Dacheng, Principles of Acupuncture and Moxibustion*. This exceptional treatise on acupuncture reinforced the principles of the *Nei Jing* and *Nan Jing* and formed the foundation for the teachings of G. Soulie de Morant, a French diplomat who devoted his middle and later years (1929 onward) to translating Chinese books, thereby introducing acupuncture practices into Europe.

▶ **1644 A.D. to 1840 A.D -** From the Qing Dynasty to the Opium Wars, herbal medicine became the main tool of physicians and, as a treatment modality, acupuncture was suppressed.

▶ **Mid 1800's -1911 A.D.** - Western Medicine was introduced into China by medical missionaries sent from Christian mission organizations. One key figure was John Kerr, an American medical missionary who arrived in Guangzhou in 1854, and remained for 47 years treating almost one million patients and training hundreds of Chinese medical students. One of his students was Sun Yat-sen, the man who later became the first president of the Republic of China.

▶ **Post Revolution of 1911 A.D.** - After the 1911 Revolution, which ended 2,000 years of imperial rule, Western medicine practices became very influential and overshadowed acupuncture. Chinese herbal medicines, as well as acupuncture, were constrained. However, due to the expanding population and need for medical care, acupuncture and herbs remained popular in rural areas giving rise to the "barefoot doctor". The barefoot doctor was usually a farmer who had received basic medical training and treated people in rural villages, attending to their basic health care.

▶ **1914 -** The Northern Warlord government proposed the abolishment of traditional Chinese Medicine, but this was strongly opposed by people using these treatments and those working in TCM all over the country.

▶ **1925 -** The Kuomingtang government succeeded in prohibiting Chinese Medicine courses from being included in medical school curriculum.

▶ **1929 -** The Kuomingtang government, through the first Congress of the Central Ministry of Health, passed a proposal entitled, "A Case for the Abolishment of the Old Medicine to Thoroughly Eliminate Public Health Obstacles". This act marked the peak of anti-Chinese Medicine sentiments. In response, throughout the country, Chinese Medicine practitioners and pharmacy workers went on strike resulting in the abandonment of the resolution. As mentioned earlier, this is also the year that acupuncture started to receive attention in Europe due to the translations of G. Soulie de Morant.

▶ **1934-1935 -** During the Long March, acupuncture was used exclusively and, despite harsh conditions, it helped maintain the health of the army. This led Mao Zedong, the leader of the Communist Party, to recognize acupuncture as an important element in China's medical system.

▶ **1950** - Chairman Mao officially united Traditional Chinese Medicine with Western Medicine and acupuncture became an established treatment in many hospitals.

▶ **1971** - Acupuncture was introduced to the mainstream in the United States through newspaper reports. Although Western medicine had been introduced into China in the early 1900s, the reverse had not happened and acupuncture and other forms of Chinese Medicine remained unknown to many people in the United States until this time.

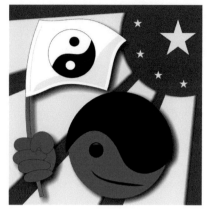

▶ **1970 to the present** - China has taken a lead role in researching all aspects of Chinese Medicine including acupuncture's application and clinical effects. Here in the U.S., acupuncture is being used and researched by many reputable organizations such as National Institutes of Health, the Military and major universities. Although the procedures of acupuncture have been modernized, it remains strongly connected to a philosophy established thousands of years ago.

I am delighted to be able share very special recollections from Kai Tao. She is the daughter of Tao Hsi-Yu (Eric HY Tao), one of the first well known acupuncturists in the U.S. In the first interview Kai has ever given about her father, she recalls his early years and the strange events that brought him to this country.

"My father, Tao Hsi-Yu was born in Beijing, China on Nov 2, 1925. His earliest exposure to acupuncture was his training as a 'barefoot doctor'. This began when he was only 14 years old. Knowing about the oppression of communist China, he snuck out of China as a teenager and wound up in England where he studied English. After several years, he migrated to Hong Kong where he worked odd jobs and finally, with permission from Taiwan, he returned to join the Navy. Although he escaped the Cultural Revolution of China, he suffered discrimination in Taiwan as a defector from China. However, in Taiwan, he had the good fortune to receive formal educational training in acupuncture and eastern medicine and proceeded to train with some of the most prominent acupuncturists in the East.

At the same time, China was opening to Western visitors and President Nixon made his first presidential trip to China with his entourage in 1971. Apparently, one of the reporters ended up requiring an emergency appendectomy which subsequently required post-operative analgesia that was effectively provided by acupuncture needles. After he returned to the U.S., the New York Times journalist shared his experience. This piqued the interest of western allopathic physicians who were learning about the utility of acupuncture for the first time. This sentinel event served as a springboard for Columbia University to invite my father to be a guest lecturer because he had a good command of the English language and was captivated by the notion of traveling west for greater opportunities.

My father, now known as Eric HY Tao, traveled extensively across the States, holding both long term didactic courses and weekend long acupuncture seminars. He worked with several medical doctors which allowed acupuncture to be guised as a legitimate service. Soon after, in 1975, he brought over the rest of his immediate family and we settled in Denver, Colorado. Acupuncture was illegal in Colorado until 1982. Thus, we have memories of my father being arrested by the police and my mom or patient supporters posting bond for his release. I recall being frightened whenever I saw a police car drive by the house because I assumed it was the police coming to arrest my father. My father worked tirelessly, seven days a week, responding to the requests of patients near and far.

Money was never an obstacle for patients because my father provided acupuncture treatment in exchange for fresh vegetables, canned foods, and baked goods. As a young girl, I recall these gifts in lieu of monetary payment as the centerpiece of our kitchen table. Growing up as a kid of an acupuncturist, my friends and acquaintances were either in awe of this mysterious field of medicine or thought my father was practicing witchcraft. I never saw a single allopathic physician from birth to 18 years old; I never missed a day of K-12 school due to sickness. Needles and herbs were the mainstay of the tools required to stay healthy in the Tao family. I recall having childhood asthma which was alleviated with herbal syrup that I took daily. This herbal concoction sat alongside my pencil box in my school backpack, akin to an inhaler. If we ever woke up sick, with no nonsense, my father would insert needles into any ailing body part and would promptly leave for work expecting either my mother or a sibling to remove the needles.

After 20 minutes, needles were removed and I was off to school. This was the norm and soon I was doing the same for my mother on a regular basis.

With unyielding harassment by law enforcement since acupuncture was still illegal in Colorado, we moved to Northern California in 1979, so that my father could start a new practice. Upon moving to California, my father's patients in Colorado and surrounding states beckoned him to return since many had reaped the health benefits of acupuncture and some were desperate for treatments that regular allopathic medicine couldn't address, especially without untoward side effects. Torn between his large patient base in the Rocky Mountain region and knowing the practice was still illegal, my father spent the next seven years flying back and forth between Colorado and California. He worked all hours, seeing patients from all walks of life, from local celebrities who wanted smoking cessation to retired race horses with chronic joint inflammation. My father never turned a single patient away. He offered house calls for oncology patients to help with pain control and nausea and worked with bedridden disabled patients for chronic problems. He was doing what he loved and patients loved what he was doing. He continued to practice for another three decades until his death in 2008. My father had two passions: 1) to insure that his children and family succeeded in the United States, and 2) to see that high quality acupuncture was accessible to all patients."

Chapter 3 - Basic Concepts In Chinese Medicine

An 'adventure' is not only exciting but it also exposes us to new experiences. In this chapter, I will provide you with 3 basic concepts that may be unusual to you but are fundamental to any discussion of Chinese Medicine. With these 3 concepts, you will be able to begin to navigate this new world of Chinese Medicine.

The 3 concepts are:

1.) Qi
2.) 5 Element Theory
3.) Yin and Yang

Qi

Qi (pronounced 'chee') is one of the essential and basic concepts in Traditional Chinese Medicine (TCM) but also one of the hardest to explain. Many people describe it as 'energy' and, while that is true, 'energy' does not capture how infinite and powerful a concept it is. Definitions taken directly from the Chinese language provide clues to understanding the meaning qi.

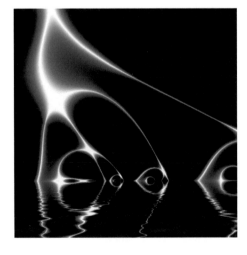

The literal translation of the Chinese character for 'health' is 'original qi.' The literal translation of the Chinese character for 'vitality' is 'high quality qi.' The literal translation of the character meaning 'friendly' is 'peaceful qi.' Why does qi appear in the translations of health, vitality, and friendliness, words that seem to be distinctly different from each other? It is because the concept of 'qi' is so basic to Chinese philosophy, it is reflected in the fundamental concepts of health, vitality, and friendliness. The Chinese are not the only people to believe in qi. Similar ideas appear in Japan as 'ki', in India as 'prana', in ancient Egypt as 'ka' and in early Greece as 'pneuma'; all of the meanings embody the idea of spirit, soul, vital spark, or essence.

You would not be alone if you wondered why, if all these cultures believe in qi and have names for it, how can 'qi' be so difficult to explain? It is, but I'll try. The commonality of all beliefs about 'qi' is that it is nonmaterial but a fundamental, essential substance that is at the core of something as large as our universe and as small as a blade of grass.

In Traditional Chinese Medicine treatments, qi is the energy that acupuncturists manipulate in order to balance your body, fight disease and help you to maintain good health. In Chinese Medicine, good health and vitality depend on sufficient amounts of qi and its ability to flow freely.

In TCM, there are distinct types of qi that your acupuncturist might mention to you. A few examples include: yuan qi (original or foundational qi); qi that is unique to a specific organ of the body (kidney qi, heart qi, etc.); and wei qi (also known as defensive qi) which guards you against invading illness. For example, if I am treating Oliver, a man who is prone to catching colds, I would consider him to be deficient in wei qi because he has a weak defense against getting sick. In Western terms, Oliver may be advised to enhance his immunity. In TCM treatment, because he is deficient or low in wei qi, I may recommend an herbal formula such as Jade Windscreen (I talk more about this formula in Chapter 5), and choose the acupuncture point Stomach 36 (a well known point to boost wei qi/immunity) to be needled. Both the herbs and acupuncture would balance Oliver's qi and help his body build up its own defenses.

5 Element Theory

The concept of the five elements appears in the very first book written about Traditional Chinese Medicine, the *Nei Jing,* which I mentioned in Chapter 2. Five Element Theory is another example of the Taoist influence on Chinese Medicine. Their belief was that human beings, as one important element in the universe, must live in harmony with the natural cycles of the environment just as plants and animals respond to and interact with the seasons. Living in unity with the seasons and the rest of our environment is a key component of health. And, because the universe is forever changing, we must continually adapt to these changes in order to remain healthy.

Classical 5 Element Theory, known in Chinese as the Wu Hsing, is based upon observations of the natural cycles of life and, in TCM, is used to interpret the relationship of the illness or wellness of your body with the natural environment. This system describes what are considered the basic 5 Elements: wood; fire; earth; metal; and water.

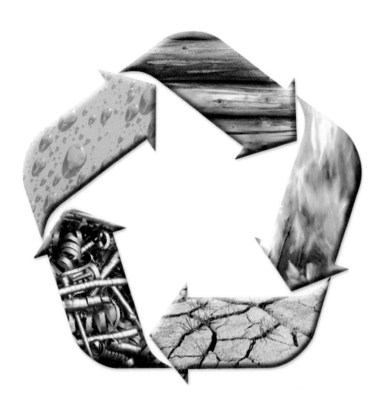

Although every one of these elements is recognizable as existing in everyday life, each one is also a metaphor or symbol designed to explain your physical and emotional relationship in the world. Each of the five elements has many things associated with it, for example a corresponding organ, color, emotion, and season of the year.

The table on the next page shows some of these correspondences. The Five Elements are listed in the column on the left and the sense organ, emotion, direction, season, taste, and color that corresponds to the particular element is in a row going from left to right.

Table Of The 5 Elements

Element	Sense Organ	Emotion	Direction	Season	Taste	Color
Wood	eyes	anger	east	spring	sour	Green /blue
Fire	tongue	joy	south	summer	bitter	Red
Earth	mouth	worry	center	late summer	sweet	Yellow
Metal	nose	grief	west	autumn	spicy	White
Water	ears	fear	north	winter	salty	black/ dark blue

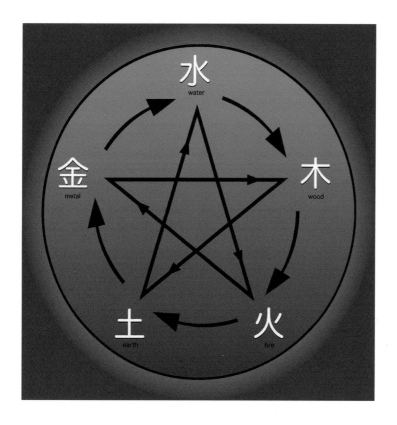

Here is one way to think about the correlation of elements to other aspects of life: Wood is the element of Spring and exemplifies the energy of growth, change and pushing through. Conversely, when thwarted or constrained, wood is also connected to emotions of frustration, anger and stress. Like the Wood element, anger can make us hard and unbendable - think of a tree that snaps in a strong wind instead of swaying. So what can we learn from the Wood element? Flexibility!

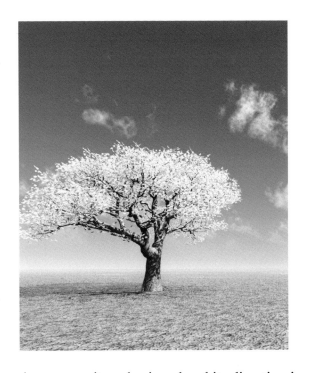

When you look at the table on the previous page, it is easy to imagine how the elements and their associations came into being so many years ago. Consider the element of Fire; its season is summer, its color is red and its direction is South, all things associated with a heat like fire. Or, look at Water; the organs associated with water have to do with bodily fluids like the kidneys and bladder, and its season is Winter which (as I know from living in Chicago) means snow which melts into water.

In the table on the next page, I show the correlation of the 5 elements to the body's organs (which are classified as either yin or yang) Notice the yang organs are all hollow organs while the yin organs are not, as in the stomach (hollow and Yang) vs. heart (solid and Yin).

Table Of The 5 Elements And Their Corresponding

Yin And Yang Organs

Element	Yin Organ	Yang Organ
Wood	liver	gallbladder
Fire	heart	small intestine
Earth	spleen	stomach
Metal	lung	large intestine
Water	kidney	urinary and bladder

Chinese Medicine, like modern medicine, recognizes that checks and balances exist within the body and in our environment. For example, if you think of checks and balances in terms of the elements, wood burns to make a fire and water can put out the flames. Now, correlate that to someone with a fever, a fire in the body. This 'fire' would benefit from colder herbs to douse the heat. TCM is exceptional because it interweaves our environment into these checks and balances through the 5 elements. Five Element Theory expresses the natural order of the universe of the universe

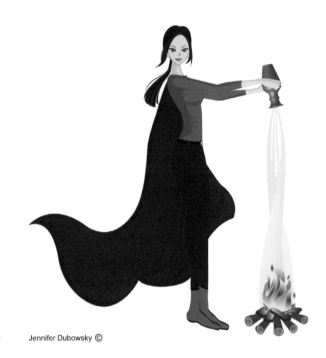

Jennifer Dubowsky ©

and our relationship to everything around us.

Yin And Yang

The concept of yin and yang is one of my favorite ideas from Chinese Medicine. Developed by the legendary sage Fu Hsu, the ideas underlying yin and yang have always struck me as extremely wise.

Today, Fu Hsu ideas are usually presented as a circular symbol such as the one below. You have probably seen this popular symbol, but many people do not know where it came from or what it represents. There are several very important ideas in this simple symbol. The first message of yin and yang is that it shows the constantly changing interactions in the universe. This is demonstrated by the dark and light flowing into and out of each other, illustrating the ebb and flow of yin and yang, light and dark, activity and rest, creation and destruction. It reminds us that everything is in motion, interrelated, and influencing our lives and nature around us. One of the best ways to understand the interrelated ideas of motion, change, and nature's influence is to remember that as soon as the sun attains its brightest glow, it begins to dim or, when we reach the top, we are also closest to beginning our descent.

The next important idea about the yin and yang concept will become clearer as you look carefully at the symbol. Do you see the dark dot in the white section of the symbol and the white dot in the black section? These dots are significant. They represent the idea that even in the most yang, there is a little yin (a tiny candle in the dark).

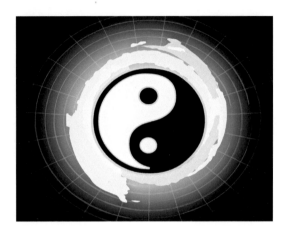

The reverse is also true. In all yin, there is the existence of a bit of yang. For example, in the most creative acts, there is a bit of destruction and in the most destructive acts, there are seeds of creation. It is inspiring to remember that there is always a small spark of hope in our darkest hour. Therefore, when we recognize that yin and yang stand for opposing forces, like dark and light or creation and destruction, we also remember that these forces are bound together, not only containing a bit of the other but also giving rise to each other. This concept lies at the heart of classic Chinese Medicine and philosophy. yin and yang demonstrates that we are all connected and interdependent.

The Difference Between Yin And Yang

In Traditional Chinese Medicine, yin and yang represent different energies, organs and bodily functions. Yin and yang also describe our relationship to the environment in which we live. They maintain opposite and equal qualities. Your healthy state, both mentally and physically is created by the right balance of yin and yang. Therefore, it is advisable to make choices from each that contribute to balance in our lives.

Yin represents a more feminine energy which endures and supports growth (think of a pregnant woman or a nursing mother). The common term "mother earth" is a good example of Yin. The earth is Yin and everything grows and receives sustenance from the earth. The table below gives some common examples of Yin.

YIN	Feminine	Night time	Dark	Cold	Earth	Calm	Contracting	Feeling	Blue

Yang, on the other hand, is masculine, generative, creative, action oriented energy. Yang develops and expands. While yin or the earth provides the nourishment, yang represents the action of growth, motion and expansion. The table below gives common examples of yang.

YANG	Masculine	Day	Light	Hot	Heaven	Active	Expanding	Thinking	Red

Yin and yang rely upon each other; they are bound together. To understand how yin and yang work together, think about blood in the human body. Blood is considered a yin fluid (nourishing) but the action that moves the blood is yang. This makes a lot of sense because we would all be in trouble if we didn't have enough blood (yin) or if it wasn't moving (yang). Another more practical example is of two people in a relationship. Pat is great at relaxing and Jody gets things done. When the balance is right and both partners are valued for their contribution, the interdependence works and everyone is happy. When the balance is off - watch out!

TCM is based on these concepts of Qi, 5 Element Theory and Yin and Yang. Each of these three concepts relies upon a fundamental understanding of the interrelatedness of living beings with their environment and the need to find an equilibrium or balance. Understanding these concepts not only gives you a clearer view of Traditional Chinese Medicine but may provide a deeper understanding of the popular discussions about creating lives of balance.

Chapter 4 - Acupuncture Adventures

What Is Acupuncture?

Acupuncture, probably the best known technique in Chinese Medicine, is the insertion of very fine needles into specific points in your body. Using this renowned technique, an acupuncturist can treat a vast variety of health concerns by promoting natural healing responses from your own body.

Acupuncture, Meridians, And Qi

The placement of needles may seem random to if you are unfamiliar with Chinese Medicine but rest assured, needles are not inserted haphazardly. To understand how acupuncture points are chosen, we have to take a short detour into the concepts of meridians. Meridians are the invisible networks that run throughout your body and provide the pathways for qi. The picture above shows a model with meridians and acupuncture points mapped out. Using the concept of meridians for thousands of years, practitioners of Traditional Chinese Medicine have mapped out the body's twelve main meridians and eight extra meridians. Each one is connected to a specific organ, or group of organs, that govern particular bodily functions. Acupuncture points are located along these meridians and when the acupuncture needle is inserted, it helps to promote the flow of qi. The stimulation of an acupoint influences the organs and functions of your body that may be distant from the area in which the needle is inserted. An acupuncture needle, inserted at the right spot, encourages your body's own healing abilities by influencing the qi. Illness results when qi is deficient, stagnates or is blocked. When qi flows freely, well-being is restored.

Needles

Many people wince at the notion of being needled and this might be a big reason why more people don't try acupuncture. This is understandable until you realize that most of today's needles have a diameter as thin as a human hair and are made of stainless steel.

It isn't anything like getting a shot at the doctor's office; I dread those. Most of my patients are pleasantly surprised by how little discomfort there is. I've included a photo so that you can see the delicacy of an acupuncture needle as compared to a human hair. I purchase needles that are pre-packaged and sterilized and dispose of them according to bio-hazard safety rules. Every practitioner I know treats needles with the same ultra-careful regard for cleanliness and health safety; you can be assured that you are being treated with clean needles and that they are only used once.

Understanding An Invisible Process

Acupuncture is both an art and a science.Previously, I described it as inserting fine needles into specific points along meridians in order to assist the free flow of qi. I know that this isn't an easy idea for those of us used to Western 'science'. I have a wonderful analogy, borrowed from Dr. Richard Tan, that will make the concepts of acupuncture, meridians and qi clearer. Imagine an overhead light (a single bulb or fancy chandelier, whatever you prefer) and now picture the switch on the wall that turns it on and off. You don't see the wires that connect the light to the switch but you feel confident that, when you flip the correct switch (the one corresponding to that particular light), the light will indeed go on. Now, apply this concept to acupuncture and meridians: Think of the light bulb

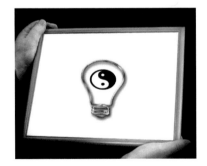

as your health problem and the switch as the needles and the wires that connect the two places as the invisible networks called meridians. When I insert the needles (flip correct switch) that link to meridians (wires running through the wall) sending qi (electric current) to reach the light bulb (your health problem) it changes the situation from dark to light.

The Balance Method Of Acupuncture

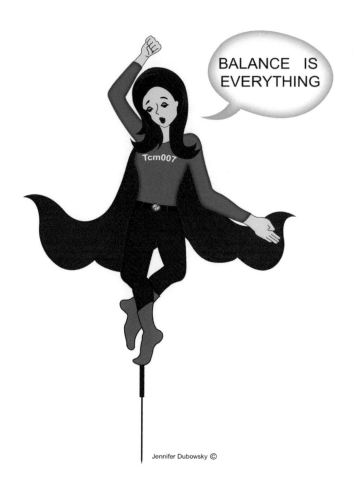

Jennifer Dubowsky ©

All acupuncture is about achieving balance, but there is more than one way to do it. I would like to briefly tell you about the Balance Method of acupuncture taught by Dr. Tan who lives and practices in San Diego, California. I consider it to be indispensable and use it regularly with very effective and speedy results. This style of acupuncture is sometimes different than what is taught in the acupuncture schools today and might be new, even to those of you who are familiar with acupuncture. The Balance Method of acupuncture uses the complicated relationships of the acupuncture meridians so that I am able to needle points on your body that are NOT in the affected area. For example, if you have ankle pain in your left foot, I would needle your right wrist. Patients are usually amazed! Often this method requires fewer needles than other methods and, when you are suffering from pain in a particular spot, you may like to have needles inserted elsewhere and still obtain relief.

30

The History Of Acupuncture

Acupuncture has been used by the Chinese and other East Asian cultures as a system of healing for over 2500 years. Needles were originally fashioned from stone or bone because that was the substance available at the time. Later, needles were made from bronze and iron, and today, stainless steel is the most common material from which needles are produced. The first written medical account of acupuncture is found in the *Nei Jing*. This classic described acupuncture, laid out the meridians, their relation to the body's organs, functions of the acupuncture points, types of qi, needling techniques, and the location of 160 acupuncture points.

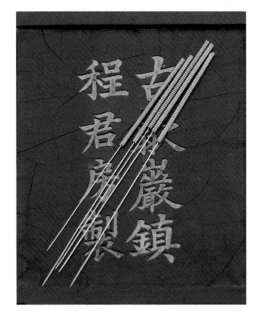

I offer you all this information, not to confuse you, but to illustrate acupuncture's long and successful Asian history before it reached the Western world in the early 1900s in France. From there, it gradually spread to other European countries but until the early 1970s, most Americans had never heard of acupuncture. That all changed with President Richard Nixon's trip to China and a reporter's emergency appendectomy in 1971. James Reston, the New York Times writer traveling with him, received acupuncture to quiet his post-operative pain. Kai Tao, in Chapter 2, refers to this event when writing about her father because Reston's subsequent stories set events in motion that changed her family's life. Reston was so impressed with the relief he experienced from acupuncture that, when he returned to the U.S., he wrote an article about it that appeared on the front page of the New York Times - introducing America to this amazing medicine! This ignited huge public interest in acupuncture. The first (mainstream) clinic, the Acupuncture Center of Washington, opened in 1972 and the news coverage was immense. Soon, hundreds of people a day came to get acupuncture treatment.

Originally there were about 20 Asian acupuncturists in D.C., and they treated over 250 patients a day. Now there are several thousand practitioners all over the country, with many schools offering Masters and Doctoral level degrees as well as hundreds of clinical studies showing the benefits of acupuncture.

Acupuncture From A Western Medical Perspective

I'm sure that, as you have been reading, you see that acupuncture, having been developed in China and other Asian cultures, has a distinctively Eastern way of looking at the healing process that is different from the more familiar Western perspective of medicine. Since it was introduced to the United States and other Western countries, teachers, writers, scientists, researchers and practitioners have attempted to reconcile the East/West differences. In hospitals and clinics, Western Medicine practitioners are now performing research experiments using 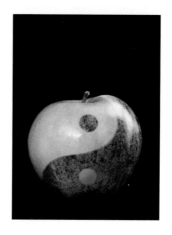 acupuncture in an effort to understand the process in Western terms. They have come up with a few theories that are not identical to Eastern thinking but don't exclude the alternative explanations. From the Western point of view, developed from numerous studies, acupuncture has been found to have the ability to alter various biochemical and physiological conditions, thereby promoting healing.

Some of the physiological effects observed by doctors in their research studies include increased circulation of blood and decreased inflammation. Pain relief has been well studied. For example, research into acupuncture's ability to reduce pain has shown that needles can cause a change in the way that the brain perceives and processes pain, thereby having a desirable effect - less pain. Studies describe how acupuncture increases the body's natural pain-killing chemicals, endorphins, which are 200 times more potent than morphine. Endorphins also affect the hormonal system and this reaction explains why acupuncture can work equally well for problems that seem to have nothing in common, such as back pain and fertility. Acupuncture has also been shown to stimulate the body to produce a chemical compound called adenosine, a painkiller your body manufactures when you are injured.

Acupuncture isn't just useful for circulation, decreased inflammation and pain relief; mental health benefits have also been found. Acupuncture regulates serotonin which has repeatedly been shown to positively affect your mood. This list briefly touches on the results from the ever-expanding Western research into the effects of acupuncture. New studies are reported daily and they add to the ever increasing body of knowledge about how acupuncture works (from a Western point of view). Articles regularly appear in mainstream journals that describe studies conducted in the best hospitals. It is important to have the effectiveness of acupuncture demonstrated in labs at top rated U.S. hospitals because experimental research will certainly lead to the treatment becoming accepted and available to everyone who wants it. If you want to read more about studies as they are published, please feel free to check my blog, Acupuncture Blog Chicago (acupuncturechicago.blogspot.com) where I provide summaries, links, and other information as it becomes available. I have also included information at the end of the book about several research studies.

Common Uses For Acupuncture

Acupuncture very successfully treats many common conditions including, but not limited to, sciatica, joint pain, migraine headaches, muscle pain, arthritis, allergies, and sinus infections. Acupuncture supports cancer treatments by reducing pain and nausea. 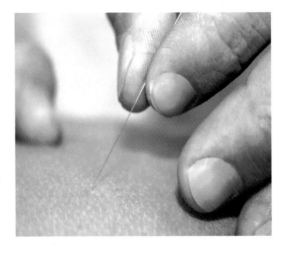 Digestive problems like diarrhea, constipation, nausea and irritable bowel syndrome respond well to acupuncture treatments. And, notably, some of the most prevalent conditions experienced by people, such as stress, depression, anxiety, PMS, fertility, PCOS, irregular menstrual periods, and menopause are all helped by these well placed needles.

Precautions And Contraindications

Acupuncture is an amazing method, very safe, and having few side effects. It is a wonderful procedure of encouraging the body to promote natural healing and improve functioning.

Side effects are unusual and luckily, problems are rare. But, there are times and conditions when I would not recommend acupuncture as your treatment. The risks mentioned below exist but are extremely uncommon.

Pregnant women are some of the best users and happiest consumers of acupuncture. Because most expectant mothers don't want to take drugs, acupuncture offers a great alternative for many of the complaints of pregnancy, including morning sickness, pain, and labor induction.

However, acupuncture in the abdominal region and in the lumbosacral area is contraindicated for pregnant women. For these women, there are also a few other points to avoid and any well trained acupuncturist will know every one of them. Don't let this warning scare you away if you are expecting; just make sure to tell your acupuncturist.

One rare adverse effect that can happen to anyone is called needle shock and it sounds worse than it is. This occurs in about 5% of acupuncture patients. They experience dizziness, nausea, or, in extreme situations, loss of consciousness. These are not lasting effects. If needle shock occurs, your practitioner will immediately remove all the needles. The majority of patients feel entirely back to normal in 10-15 minutes and suffer no ongoing consequences.

Overall, as the National Institutes of Health conclude, acupuncturists have an extremely good safety record. Generally, the most common risk of having an acupuncture treatment is getting a bruise at the needle site.

One effect that I tell my patients about, although it doesn't happen often, is that their original symptoms could feel worse for a couple of hours or days after an acupuncture treatment. This is similar to some reactions after a massage – soreness before you feel better.

It is also possible that, during the treatment, you might feel emotional and cry or laugh. Don't worry, you won't be the first or last patient to have emotions evoked by the process. All these reactions are common and should not cause concern but always discuss your experiences with your acupuncturist during the visit and call her if you have any concerns after a treatment. Your comfort and well being are always a top priority. The more you communicate with your acupuncturist, the more she will be able to help you.

One Patient's Recollection Of Her First Treatment

One of my patients, a woman in her fifties who has lived with chronic rheumatoid arthritis for more than 25 years, recalled her first acupuncture treatment.

"When I made my first acupuncture appointment, the potential for relief from the constant pain of rheumatoid arthritis (RA) forced me to overcome a life-long fear of needles. The incredible outcome from that first visit caused me to immediately sign-up for another treatment. While there is no cure for RA, the Balance Method of acupuncture offers respite from pain as well as a sense of well-being and balance, all without the significant side effects of prescribed pharmaceuticals. Initially, I did not understand or care why a needle in my ankle would cause my shoulder pain to disappear but, as I continued to receive acupuncture, I became an active participant in my own treatments. When a particular series of needles left me feeling pain-free for days, I made sure to report that at my next treatment.

There are different series of needles and points that can be used to relieve specific pain or address a lack of energy, as well as feelings of anxiety or stress. Having a long-term relationship with an acupuncturist allows us to build on established successes as well as experimenting with new techniques that she learns in her continuing education seminars."

Chapter 5 - Herbs

Herbal Medicine refers to the use of plants, flowers, minerals and animal sources for healing. When we talk about Chinese Herbal Medicine, we are talking about a sophisticated form of treatment that has been around much longer than Western pharmaceuticals, not only in

China, but in many parts of the world. When I was completing my training with an internship in Beijing, China, (that's me in the photo, with one of the doctors) I studied at the Sino-Friendship Hospital, a Western

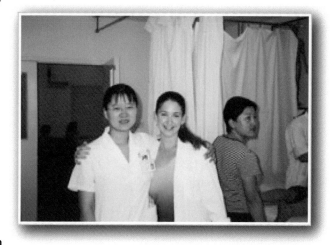

hospital that had a full herbal pharmacy. This well stocked pharmacy was in addition to the Western style dispensary. Herbal pharmacies are not unusual in China, but hospitals are not the only place to locate good quality herbs. Local shops and remedies are widespread, popular, and integral to the culture.

During the last several years in this country and all over the world, we have witnessed a resurgence of interest in the use of natural ingredients. The increased interest in herbs in the U.S. is only one element of a greater movement toward finding healthy, alternative solutions to life's problems. The increased attention to 'natural', 'green' and 'organic' can be seen in cosmetics, clothing, architecture, and especially in food and food supplements. It makes sense, of course, to look to health solutions that are closer to nature, have fewer side effects than pharmaceutical drugs, and are often less expensive.

How Is Chinese Herbal Medicine Different From Western Herbal Medicine?

There are many traditional Chinese formulas and each one is prepared using a careful balance of herbs. Your licensed Chinese Medicine practitioner will decide upon the formula best suited to you and it may have as many as 20 different herbs, unlike Western herbal medicine which tends to use one or two herbs to treat a specific symptom. Chinese Medicine formulas are selected for you based on your unique symptoms, medical history and your body's constitution. The next section further explains how herbs and formulas are chosen specifically for your needs.

Choosing Herbs

Your TCM practitioner is the best person to rely on when choosing Chinese herbs, but I do want you to be familiar with types of herbs so that you have a better understanding of how your practitioner makes her choices. Herbs are highly specific in their actions, possess diverse qualities, and have properties that target different aspects of an ailment. The major classifications of herbs include, but are not limited to: hot or cold, bitter or sweet, and drying or moist. Therefore, in striving to

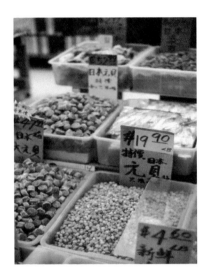

balance your body, when your illness is warmer in nature, cooling herbs are the appropriate remedy and would be suggested. Or, if you were experiencing a dry cough, your practitioner is likely to choose herbs that moisten your throat. Let's look more specifically at an ordinary sickness - the common cold. The cold is usually an illness with a warmer nature and has heat signs, such as a thick yellow tongue coating, fever, sweating, yellow phlegm and a sore throat. When that is the case, your herbal formula is likely to include herbs of a colder nature to cool the

heat in your body and drying herbs in order to clear out the phlegm. If however, you were experiencing the chills, had a thick white coating, no fever and clear phlegm, warmer herbs would be the more appropriate choice.

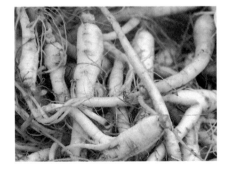

Another common problem that responds well to herbal medicine is premenstrual syndrome or PMS. When a woman experiences cramps, irritability and bloating prior to her menstrual period, it is because of stagnation (commonly called 'blood stagnation') so blood moving herbs would be recommended. If bloating is her main concern, then the formula might also include herbs to drain damp (excess fluid) from her body. From these simple examples, you can see how herbal formulas have to be specifically tailored to the needs of each patient and your presenting problem.

I don't want you to think of herbs only as an answer for colds, pains and illnesses. Herbs are not just for those times when you are in trouble, so don't wait until you feel miserable to consider using them. Herbs are also very effective in maintaining your health and keeping your body in balance. For example, Jade Windscreen, the formula I mentioned in the section on qi, is a popular and classic formula with a well-deserved reputation for boosting your immune system. The history of Jade Windscreen goes back 1000 years in China where it has been effective for people who are prone to colds, flus, and allergies. It is also a great preventative formula if you are traveling, flying or have been exposed to sick people. If you have a chronic problem, like insomnia, depression, or ongoing allergies, once you feel better it might still be in your best interest to keep taking herbs regularly, at least for a period of time. This will help to maintain the herbs' good results and hopefully prevent the old problem from returning or a new one from forming.

The History Of Chinese Herbal Medicine

Long, long before the big drug boom, herbal remedies were widely used to treat people's complaints and to help them maintain wellness. In China, the first record of herbs appeared in the previously mentioned *Yellow Emperor's Classic of Internal Medicine* which listed 28 herbal substances and 12 prescriptions. Around that same time, a friend of the Yellow Emperor, Shen Nong, lived in the great Yellow River Plateau and was well known for his agricultural advancements.

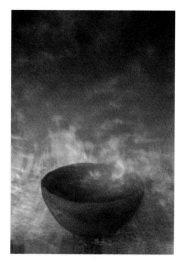

He wrote the classic book, *Materia Medica* also known as *Shen Nong Ben Cao Jing* or *The Divine Farmer's Materia Medica* (Shen Nong can be translated as Divine Farmer). He was also reputed to have ingested many substances in order to test their effects first hand, which may have been how he died. In all, he recorded around 365 healing substances and also warned practitioners which herbs could be toxic. *The Divine Farmer's Materia Medica* laid the foundation for the study of Chinese medicinals and was the first text to discuss the properties of herbs as we do now: hot, cold, dry, moist, and more.

Much later, around 220 A.D., Jiang Zhongjing, a doctor, wrote the *Shang Han Lun*, a very famous classical text that is still in publication today. I have a copy in English. This book about Chinese Herbal Medicine contains 200 formulas and treatment based on pattern discrimination.

In 659 A.D., the Revised *Materia Medica* contained illustrations of herbs and 844 entries. It was revised again in 1108 A.D., and, in that edition of more than fifteen hundred entries, herbs were arranged according to patterns. The final revision in 1596 A.D., further expanded the *Materia Medica* to almost nineteen hundred entries. Today, the *Materia Medica* is still being further refined as additional clinical and scientific data becomes available.

The interest and expansion of herbal knowledge did not stop with the *Materia Medica*. There are always individuals, scientists and lay people, who want to learn newer ways of using natural ingredients. In 1977, the *Encyclopedia of Traditional Chinese Medicinal Substances* listed 5767 herbs and formulas. You can see that the art and science of herbal medicine is vibrant and continues to evolve. Practitioners of both Western and Eastern medicine continue to research and learn more about restoring and maintaining health by using herbs.

Selecting Quality Herbs

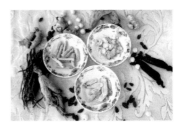

It is important to know what to look for when you purchase herbs. If you follow the recommendation of your acupuncturist or herbalist, she will already have done this work for you. However, when you select herbs on your own, you want to be sure that you chose herbs of the highest potency, quality, and safety.

Like most practitioners, I always order from companies that are Good Manufacturing Practice (GMP) certified. A GMP certification means that the manufacturer has met consistent and controlled quality standards and the products have been evaluated by an independent inspector.

Sometimes you can find GMP certified herbs in stores but many of these companies will only sell to health care providers. Herbs, unlike chemically made drugs, are not under the control of the U.S. Food and Drug Administration so it becomes even more important to be responsible in your selection or, better yet, rely on an expert's advice.

Herbs come in many forms including herbal teas, liquid extracts, pills, granules, creams and salves. When used correctly under the guidance of your TCM practitioner, herbs are generally safe and rarely have side effects. You can often combine ordinary Western drugs with Chinese herbs, but there are exceptions, particularly in the case of blood thinners such as Coumadin. To be safe, you need to always tell your Western doctor what herbs you are taking and tell your acupuncturist or herbalist which chemical drugs you take. If you do notice any side effects, please stop taking your herbs and consult your herbalist right away. Also, if you are going to be having a surgical procedure, I suggest you stop all herbs two weeks prior to surgery.

Chinese Herbal Medicine is not only very old and exotic, but it is also a highly complex and useful form of medicine for a wide range of complaints and everyday health concerns. As with any substance that has the capability of affecting your body, herbs need to be taken seriously.

Your Own Herbal Pharmacy

Many people keep an herbal cabinet in their homes so they have easy access to formulas that they use frequently. I certainly keep a supply of herbs at home but I am careful not to stock too many because the formulas must be fresh. If you want to build an herbal supply, I have provided some ideas below but remember to discard herbs when they expire.

Here are the names and uses for herbs that might find their way into your own herbal pharmacy.

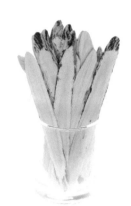

Huang qi/Astragalus - I have written about this herb many times on my blog and with good reason. Astragalus contains antioxidants which stimulate the immune system. It is also anti-inflammatory and antibacterial. Therefore, astragalus is often used to treat and prevent the common cold, sinus infections, allergies and other upper respiratory infections. This is one of the few Chinese herbs that are used in formulas and as a single herb. Astragalus is available in capsules, tablets and teas. Astragalus tea, which is made from the dried root of the astragalus plant can be bought in some stores or ordered online. You can also make astragalus tea in your own kitchen by boiling and then simmering the dried root.

Yin Qiao (also spelled Yin Chiao) - This Chinese herbal formula is a great first line of defense against the common cold. It is best taken at the initial signs of a cold or flu, especially if you have a sore throat. If you take it soon enough, you might prevent the illness. If it is too late for prevention, you will have lessened the duration and severity of the cold. Most Chinese herbal practitioners carry this formula but it can also be found in some grocery stores such as Whole Foods.

Ginger Tea - Ginger tea is probably my most frequent recommendation of an herbal remedy to keep at home because it is good for so many things. Ginger acts as an anti-inflammatory so it is good for pain relief and other inflammatory conditions. It is also excellent for the digestive system, especially nausea and can be safely used for morning sickness. I also recommend it for PMS and for enhancing fertility because it is warming to the middle region of your body. Like astragalus, you could simmer up some tea in your home but ginger tea is not hard to find in stores. My favorite brand is by Traditional Medicinals, a company that produces many fine teas.

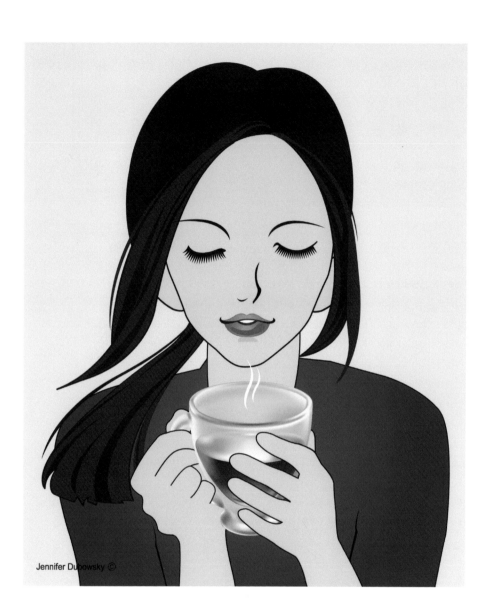

Jennifer Dubowsky ©

Chapter 6 – Cupping

In previous chapters, I described acupuncture and herbal medicines, the best known and most popular treatments in the practice of Traditional Chinese Medicine. In this chapter, I will explain cupping. Many people are unfamiliar with cupping although it did gain momentary fame when actress Gwyneth Paltrow walked a red carpet wearing a glamorous strapless gown with purple cupping circles apparent on her back. "I 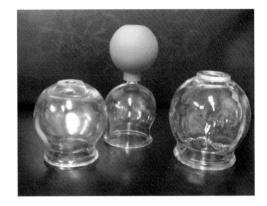 have been a big fan of Chinese medicine for a long time because it works," Paltrow told reporters who wondered about the odd circles on her back. Since then, Victoria Beckham, Jessica Simpson and Denise Richards have all shown off their tell tale cupping marks.

What Is Cupping?

Cupping is a common and highly effective treatment used in Traditional Chinese Medicine. This technique involves a skilled practitioner carefully placing sterile glass, bamboo or plastic jars (they often look like jelly jars) on particular areas of your skin. The cups come in various sizes and you can see an example of common cups in the photo above..

Your Chinese Medicine practitioner will suction the air out of each cup in order to create a vacuum. As she proceeds, she will ask about your comfort and you will determine the intensity of the suction. The result is that the underlying tissue is raised, or sucked, part way into the cup. Cupping can help detox toxins from the body and stimulate the flow of fresh blood, lymph, and qi to the affected area of your body.

You can see the raised skin under the cup in the photo on the next page. As the suction draws your skin upward, you will usually feel a tight sensation in the area of your body under the cup. This pull generally feels good and relaxing for your aching muscles.

Your practitioner can create suction in the cup in one of several different ways. One method, an older, traditional technique, involves swabbing rubbing alcohol onto the bottom of a glass cup, lighting it with a flame, and then putting the cup quickly

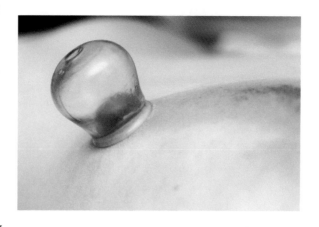

against the skin. When this method is used, flames are never allowed near your skin. Fire is the means to create enough heat to produce suction inside the cups. You can see an example of fire cupping on the next page.

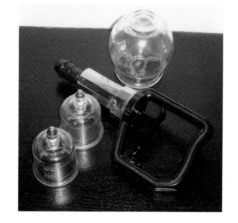

To the right, I've included a photo of a more modern set of cups. I often use these in my acupuncture practice. They have a small pump especially designed for the purpose of suction. The pump works gently, can be controlled, and does not involve fire. Another advantage to this more modern version is that the amount of suction is easily adjustable to your comfort.

One very common area to be cupped is your back. My patients have often told me how relaxing cupping is on their backs. Other areas of your body, such as your limbs and buttocks, can be successfully cupped; the fleshy parts of your body are the preferred sites. The cups are generally left in place for 5-20 minutes, depending on your comfort and your practitioner's assessment of your problem.

There are usually colored circles or streaks (depending on the cupping method) that remain after the cups are removed. I always warn patients in advance that cupping will turn their skin temporarily red, blue or purple, similar to an 'acupuncture hickey'.

This is normal, especially if there is an energetic blockage under the cups, but if my patients want to avoid any chance of bruising, we do not use this procedure.

Gwynth Paltrow can make a fashion statement with cupping marks but other people are reluctant to be seen in a swimsuit or gown with colorful marks on their back. The skin discoloration can 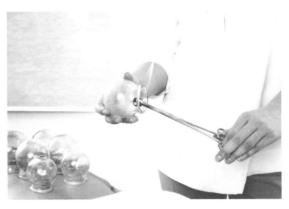 last anywhere from a few days to a couple of weeks but it causes no discomfort. Occasionally a patient will report a sense of soreness similar to having had a deep tissue massage. Rarely, blisters will appear but they are painless and are naturally reabsorbed into the skin within a few days.

One way to think about cupping is that it is the inverse of massage. Rather than applying pressure to muscles, the suction uses mild pressure to pull skin, tissue and muscles upward. I often combine cupping with acupuncture in one treatment, but it can also be used alone. Once the marks have cleared, the procedure can be repeated until the condition is resolved.

Methods Of Cupping

Some styles of cupping are used more commonly than others but there are a number of methods, including: **Fixed Cupping; Moving Cupping; Needle Cupping; Flash Cupping** and **Bleeding Cupping**. The various methods may use cups of assorted sizes and different strengths of suction, depending on what is needed. Here is a very brief explanation of each.

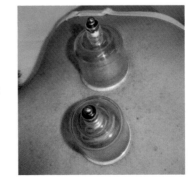

Fixed Cupping - The cups are placed on a selected area of your body and left in place without being moved. You can see an example to your right, in the photo.

Moving Cupping - As the name implies, in this method your practitioner applies massage oil or cream on your skin in selected places, puts the cups over the areas to be treated and slides them around that region of your body, usually your back. The cups slide easily because the cream has lubricated your body.

Needle Cupping - Cups are sometimes placed over an acupuncture needle that has been inserted. They are left in place and not moved, they don't touch the needle.

Flash Cupping - In this method, your practitioner applies a cup for a very short period of time and removes it.

Bleeding Cupping - Bleeding cupping is an older method, very uncommon in the U.S., but it can be effective. During a regular cupping session, a little blood might be drawn up once in awhile, especially if the cup is placed over the spot where a needle had been inserted. In Bleeding Cupping, a sterile surgical instrument is used to scrape the skin and the cup is then applied.

Contraindications And Cautions

Many of my patients look forward to cupping in conjunction with their acupuncture treatments because it is so effective in relieving certain problems but, everyone is different, so be sure to share any health conditions or personal concerns with your practitioner. In my practice, if a patient is new to cupping, I usually make the first cupping session shorter to see how they respond to the treatment before lengthening the amount of time I leave cups on the body. There are reasons to avoid cupping. If you have a skin irritation or an open wound, that area should not be cupped. If you have skin ulcers or edema, also avoid cupping. If you are pregnant, your practitioner will use extreme caution and never allow cupping on your abdomen or lower back. Everybody else, enjoy the sensation and the results.

The History Of Cupping

Although most people think of Traditional Chinese Medicine when they hear about cupping, similar treatment techniques have evolved in many other cultures. Cupping therapy is believed to have been used 3,500 years ago in Egypt. Pictographs and hieroglyphic writings that have been unearthed in certain regions have led researchers to these conclusions.

In ancient Greece, Hippocrates (460-370 BC), a man who many consider to be the 'Father of Modern Medicine' discussed both wet and dry cupping in his guide to clinical treatment. He recommended the use of cups for a variety of ailments, including angina, menstrual irregularities and other disorders.

In China, the earliest use of cupping was recorded by the famous Taoist, alchemist and herbalist, Ge Hong (281–341 A.D.) in an ancient tract called the *Handbook of Prescriptions for Emergencies*. He was famous as an accomplished healer and trusted confidante of many high officials in ancient China. During those times, Ge Hong and other medicine men used animal horns for cups. That is why some medical

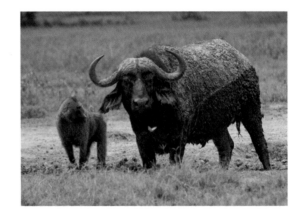

descriptions refer to cupping as the 'horn method' of healing. The use of horns was not confined to China. In Europe, other areas of Asia, Africa and North America, animal horns were hollowed out, fashioned into effective cups and used for treatment of many ailments. No one was ordering sets of cups on the Internet - they used natural resources. For example, natives along the west coast of North America used shells. Further south, the natives made their cupping implements by slicing off the point of a buffalo horn. They would then place the base of the horn on the body, stuff grass in the top and light it on fire to create a vacuum. Primarily, the horn was used to remove thorns and withdraw pus or illness from the body. Another technique used to withdraw disease was to suck air through a hollowed bone tube, to create suction like a drinking straw.

Cupping remained in use both in China and throughout Europe and was practiced by well known physicians such as Paracelsus (1493-1541) and Ambroise Pare (1509-1590). In 1826, surgeon Charles Kennedy wrote, "The art of cupping has been so well-known, and the benefits arising from it so long experienced, that it is quite unnecessary to bring forward testimonials in favor of what has received not only the approbation of modern times, but also the sanction of remotest antiquity".

There was a decline of its use in the mid 1800's, but cupping enjoyed a bit of a revival in the early 1900's. In the last few decades, its effectiveness as a treatment has improved cupping's popularity here in the U.S. In China, extensive research has been carried out on cupping, and the practice is a mainstay of government-sponsored hospitals of Traditional Chinese Medicine (TCM). The fundamental therapeutic value of cupping has been documented through several thousand years of clinical and subjective experience.

When Is Cupping Indicated?

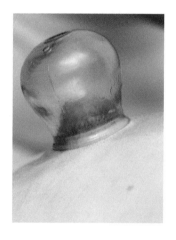

Cupping is indicated to warm and promote the free flow of qi and blood in the meridians (if you want to refresh your memory about qi and meridians, please refer back to Chapter 3 and the definitions provided at the beginning of the book). It is used to improve energy and blood flow throughout your body and to specific areas. The vacuum created by cupping draws up the non-circulating, stagnant blood and fluids from the affected area, bringing them to the surface so that healthy, unobstructed circulation can be restored. Cupping provides pain relief, loosens muscles, pulls toxins out of your body and can be incredibly relaxing.

Common conditions that respond well to cupping include: back and neck pain; stiff muscles; anxiety; fatigue; migraines; rheumatism; certain skin conditions; colds and allergies; and even digestive disorders. This treatment is valuable for your lungs and can clear congestion from a common cold or bronchitis; it helps to control asthma. In fact, respiratory conditions are one of the most common maladies that cupping is used to relieve. This ancient and innovative method has been proven effective against many common disorders. I commonly use it in my practice with great results and find that the majority of my patients who receive cupping therapy really like it and find it helpful in their over all wellness as well as relief from specific concerns.

Common Questions About Cupping (and answers)

Q. Does Cupping hurt?

A. Generally cupping does not hurt. Cups may feel tight or pinch you slightly when they are first applied but the suction level is adjustable. Therefore, if the cups feel too tight, you can ask your practitioner to reduce the amount of suction.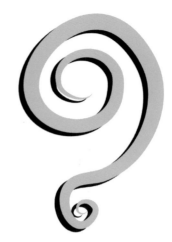

Q. Would you Cup me each time I come to your office?

A. That would depend on how far apart your appointments are. Often, your practitioner will wait until most of the color/bruises from your previous cupping session have cleared up, or gotten significantly lighter, before offering you more cupping.

Q. Do you always use the cups on my back?

A. The back is the most common place on the body to receive cupping but it can be done elsewhere, generally on the fleshy areas of your body.

Q. You would never cup my face, would you?

A. I don't, but it is done. However, face cupping is not common in the United States because many patients do not like the idea of a bruised complexion, an understandable concern.

Chapter 7 - Moxabustion

What Is Moxabustion?

Moxabustion, often called 'moxa', is another popular treatment in Traditional Chinese Medicine and can be used alone or in conjunction with acupuncture. The term moxa is derived from the Japanese 'mogusa' referring to the herb named mugwort and the Latin 'bustion' meaning burning and that is exactly what moxabustion is all about - burning mugwort on

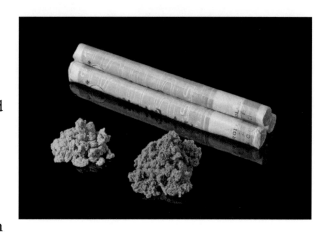

or near your skin. Mugwort is a close relative of the beautiful and prized chrysanthemum flower. The finished product that you will see in your acupuncturist's office has been made from the spongy, wooly substance found in a certain variety of the plant. The material is shaped into different forms. A couple of examples are in the photo above. Your acupuncturist selects the size and shape of moxa depending on the particular moxabustion technique that she intends to use. The commonality in all moxa treatments is that heat is created by burning the moxa and applying it either directly or indirectly to the skin.

Moxa Techniques: Moxabustion is used either as indirect moxa or direct moxa. Most acupuncturists, including myself, do **not** use direct moxa.

Indirect Moxa Techniques

All of the techniques involve burning a piece of moxa close enough to your skin to produce heat but at a safe enough distance to prevent any possibility of hot material touching your body.

1. Moxa Stick - A moxa stick is shaped like a cigar. You can see a photo of a stick to the right. It is lit and held an inch or two away from your skin to stimulate an acupuncture point or points.

Another way to use a moxa stick is to move it around above the appropriate area of the body. A common place for this technique is the abdomen. The moxa stick can also be used after needles have been placed in your body. Your practitioner may touch the moxa stick to the needle to further warm and stimulate the point. In my Chicago practice, I will often show patients who I think would benefit from moxa, how to use a moxa stick on their own so they can enhance their treatments by using the stick (without needles) at home.

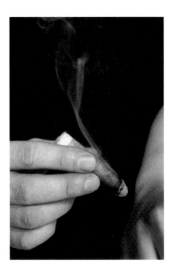

2. Needle Top Moxa - Your acupuncturist may place a small piece of moxa on the top of an acupuncture needle and heats the moxa. The heat warms the needle but does not burn you. You will feel a pleasant warming sensation at the point.

3. A Belly Bowl - Belly bowls are small containers that hold burning moxa. The bowl is placed directly above the belly button, hence the name. In this method, a piece of ginger or garlic is placed between your skin and belly bowl. Again, you do not have to worry about being burned with this or any of the other techniques.

4. Stick-on Moxa - In fact, many companies sell moxa that comes with a built in shield to further protect you. So, you can moxa directly on a point and still be safe because there is a barrier between the moxa and the skin. The photo to the right is an example of stick on moxa.

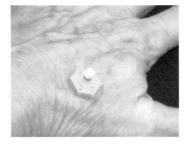

The purpose of the different moxa techniques is to bring a pleasant warm sensation to the area of skin around the appropriate points. Your practitioner will usually continue burning the moxa until your skin becomes pinkish and she will always adjust the intensity of the heat to keep you comfortable while getting the best effect.

Direct Moxa

Direct moxa is a rarely used technique in the U.S. because it involves burning a piece of moxa on a specific acupuncture point on your skin. Not surprisingly, this approach is less common than indirect techniques because there is a much higher risk of burning your skin when moxa is placed directly on the surface area.

Conditions For Which Moxabustion Is Used

Moxibustion therapy can be effective for many diseases and conditions, particularly those problems that Chinese Medicine considers cold or stagnant in nature. Some of the main disorders treated with moxa include: asthma; diarrhea; rheumatic pain; abdominal pain; vomiting; certain digestive disorders; arthritis; back pain; muscle stiffness; anxiety; and female health problems such as menstrual cramps, irregular periods, and infertility; and any kind of pain due to cold or deficiency. Moxabustion can also be an effective tool in turning breach babies when it is used on a point near the pinky toe. I have had great success with this simple treatment for pregnant women.

Moxa works by helping to warm the meridians, open channels, regulate qi and blood flow in your body, expel cold and dampness and, for women, warm your uterus.

Contraindications

Moxa should not be used if you have been diagnosed with a heated constitution or illness. For example, moxa would not be appropriate for someone with a high fever. It also should not be used over irritated skin or open wounds.

The History Of Moxabustion

Moxabustion was developed in the north region of China, where the weather is cold and dry. It originated as humans began to find uses for fire. One theory is, that while warming themselves by the fire, ancient humans accidentally found relief from pain or illness when certain areas of their skin were warmed by heat. From that, they learned to use ignited branches or hay to warm the pained or ill parts of their bodies.

Eventually, knowing the varieties of herbs and flowers, mugwort was found to be ideal for this purpose because it is easily ignited and produces a mild heat.

In the Middle Ages, mugwort gained popularity because people believed it was a magical herb that could protect travelers against evil spirits and wild animals. This myth may have gotten started because mugwort was effective in repelling insects, especially moths, from gardens. The repellant properties may have been exaggerated as stories were told over time, changing insect resistance to warding off evil spirits. Another tale is that Roman soldiers put mugwort in their sandals to protect their feet against fatigue.

The ancient stories may be fanciful, but it is true that moxibustion techniques have been refined and the uses of burning moxa continue to be developed, providing many benefits.

A good friend and fellow acupuncturist, Nicole Hohman, L.A.c., talks about her experiences using moxabustion.

"In my practice I use moxa most often for menstrual pain, strengthening digestive function, and fatigue, but I also use it for turning breech babies and for curing bedwetting in children.

One case in which moxa was very helpful, was for a 10 year old girl who came to me for treatment for her Crohn's disease, an inflammatory bowel disease that creates pain and diarrhea and ulcers in the intestines. She was underweight for her age and her symptoms were not under control despite taking medications. Her energy was low, she had a pale tongue and pale complexion which indicated Qi deficiency. Not surprisingly, her situation would be difficult for anyone but especially stressful for a child. She also had a lot of anxiety about going to school and having urgent diarrhea in school so she would stay home many mornings when her symptoms were at their worst. We began acupuncture and moxa and, in the first few weeks, her stomach pain and diarrhea improved and she began to feel calmer. After three months into the treatment course, she had a growth spurt and missed much less school because of anxiety and her Crohn's symptoms.

Correcting breech presentation with moxa is safe, painless and cost effective compared to the manual version or the eventual cesarean section that women may need if the baby doesn't turn by itself, so it is always a pleasure when a woman with breech presentation shows up on my schedule. A study in the Journal of the American Medical Association found moxa for breech presentation to be

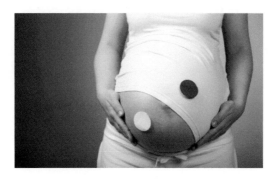

more than 80% effective. A 33 year old woman came to me when she was 35 weeks pregnancy with a breech fetus. I performed the moxa and taught her and her husband how to continue the treatments on their own at home for 20 minutes twice a day. I gave them a few sticks of moxa and asked them to return to the clinic if there was no change in two weeks. A week and a half later she called to tell me the baby had turned."

Chapter 8 - Tui na

Tui na (pronounced "twee nah") is a form of Asian bodywork that is the oldest known system of massage. It translates literally as 'push and grasp' in Chinese and is an important modality in TCM treatments. Like several of the other modalities I have discussed, tui na techniques were described in The Yellow Emperor's *Classics of Internal Medicine.*

Tui na is different from a Swedish or deep tissue massage, two types of massage commonly practiced in the U.S. First of all, during tui na, you are dressed in your own comfortable clothing and are seated in a chair or lying on a massage table. The practitioner not only uses her hands on your arms, legs and back but also employs her elbows and knees in a variety of manipulations that include compression, pressing, kneading and tapping. There are some similarities between tui na and acupressure (using pressure instead of needles on acupuncture points) because the goals of both treatments are to stimulate acupoints during the massage. Your practitioner's intention is to encourage the flow of qi, rebalance energy and, of course, to help you to feel your best.

Indications For The Use Of Tui na

Tui na is helpful with a variety of complaints, including: neck pain; back pain; muscle pain; constipation; PMS; and other conditions where body manipulation can be very effective.

Often tui na sessions are vigorous so you may not find it to be as relaxing as other forms of massage. There is certainly stronger and more active work on the part of the tui na massage therapist than is commonly experienced when you have a spa massage. Some patients feel sore after a session but that doesn't usually last long. Tui na is used medically in hospitals in China where practitioners manipulate your body in order to free up blocked energy as well as to loosen tight joints and muscles.

Contraindications

If patients suffer from certain conditions, I advise them to avoid tui na. Problems such as osteoporosis or conditions involving fractures dictate passing up tui na. Also, if you have an infectious disease, skin problem, or an open wound, stay away from this type of massage.

I have benefited from tui na and consider it a valuable tool. However I am not a gifted tui na practitioner so I refer to others if a condition requires tui na or if patient is interested in trying this type of massage. With that in mind, I am including the experience of Diane Lowry, L.A.c., who is an accomplished tui na therapist in Richmond, Virginia. I have included a photo of Diane performing tui na.

"In my practice, I use Tui na as both a diagnostic tool and as a treatment method. Direct contact along the channels and at specific acupuncture points provides insight into the nature of the patient's condition – whether their underlying pattern is excess or deficient, how their body responds to light versus firm pressure, and how easily their body releases stress and tension.

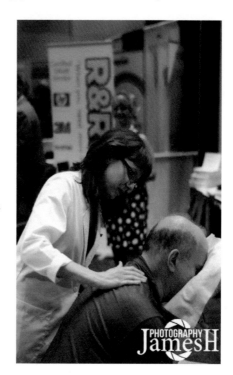

Sharing tui na has been a fantastic way for me to connect more deeply with my patients. As I follow each breath cycle and focus my attention on subtle changes in his or her body, I must be fully present and aware. This mindfulness of the present moment, coupled with setting my intention for their highest good, has had been lovely way of healing both the patient and myself."

Chapter 9 – Pattern Diagnosis

Chinese healers of 2500 years ago had to detect the internal problems of your body from external clues. To do this, they developed unique and functional diagnostic tools that have withstood the test of time. Many of today's practices, including pattern diagnosis, are refinements of techniques created long ago.

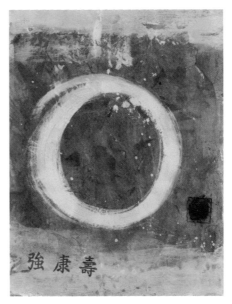

To understand the evolution of pattern diagnosis, imagine that you are consulting a Chinese doctor in the year 400 B.C.E. He cannot see inside your body and has no scans or X-ray machines to show him the cause of your complaints. So, the wise doctor must figure out what is going on internally from what he observes and what you, as the patient, tell him about your symptoms. He asks questions and uses the other tools available to him. After he assembles the information, he diagnoses your illness, but he must explain the problem in a language that makes sense to both of you. Perhaps you have the condition we now call a fever. Because you and your doctor understand your description of a fever as being similar to fire (a familiar element in 400 B.C.E), it is reasonable to think about your disease as a 'hot' disease. Twenty-five hundred years ago in China, he may have explained it to you as a problem of 'excess heat'. When we place ourselves in that era, it becomes very reasonable to see how these familiar elements from the environment (hot, cold, wind, damp) were used to describe ailments that exist in the human body. Everyone could understand the terms because everyone would have respected and been knowledgeable about the forces of nature such as wind, rain, and sun. If this sounds odd to you, remember that natural elements are mighty and can have tremendous effects on our lives. We have not forgotten Hurricane Katrina, the wildfires in the West and the storm Sandy that demolished parts of the East coast. Natural elements are so much a part of our common vocabularies that we even use them in reference to our friends and family all the time.

For example: 'she's a cold fish', 'he has a hot temper', 'he gave me an icy stare', or 'she's hot'. See what I mean?

Pattern diagnosis describes your symptoms in terms of imbalances in your body and uses terms from nature such as hot, cold, damp, dry, wind and Chinese words, like yin and yang. Even if these descriptions seem unusual to us today, we can appreciate that pattern diagnosis was in keeping with the prevailing philosophy of the time: to be healthy, it is important that we live in harmony with our world and "go with the flow".

In pattern diagnosis, each pattern represents a set of symptoms and observations about a patient. There are numerous patterns of disharmony, a few common examples have names like Liver Qi stagnation, Spleen Qi deficiency or Kidney yin deficiency. How does your practitioner detect the pattern you are experiencing? Using the tools below, she can identify the pattern (or patterns) and create a treatment plan to return your body to a balanced, more vibrant state of health.

The Fundamental Tools Of Chinese Medicine

The fundamental tools of TCM are: asking you **questions** about your body, lifestyle, and emotions; **observation of your face and body; tongue diagnosis;** and **pulse diagnosis**. This leads to identification of any patterns of disharmony.

▶ **Questions**

Asking questions is an obvious technique for gathering information and is a genuine skill. Many patients who have spent time in Western medical offices complain that their doctor failed to ask the right questions, or worse, failed to be interested enough to ask enough questions. Your TCM practitioner will ask you to fill out paperwork and then she will follow up with numerous questions about your health and lifestyle; some may surprise you. A few examples: Do you wake up during the night? Do you have regular bowel movements? Is your menstrual cycle regular? How is your energy level? Do you eat a lot of spicy or cold foods? These are not random questions. Your answers help your practitioner to begin to understand your unique strengths and imbalances.

► **Observation Of Your Face And Body**

We observe other people everyday and, without always realizing it, we pick up clues to their health, emotions, and well being. Even without exchanging words, you might notice a friend's sad posture, shallow breathing, or a painful facial expression. You didn't need to be trained to wonder if something was wrong. When your TCM practitioner observes your face and body, she checks obvious signs and a great deal more. A few things I might notice are: discolorations of your skin and where the poor color is located; dark circles under your eyes; and bloating in any area of your body. I will ask myself, does this person emanate vitality? I will make a note of your posture and body type. Again, these observations and others are just the beginning but they contribute to understanding your body's messages and identifying any patterns of disharmony.

The two tools described previously - questions and observations of your face and body - may be pursued more deeply in Eastern treatment than in Western offices but they are familiar. The next two diagnostic tools are unique to Chinese Medicine.

► **Tongue Diagnosis**

Tongue diagnosis is just what is sounds like - a visual inspection of your tongue in order to gain information about your well-being. Practitioners of TCM (Traditional Chinese Medicine) consider it to be an essential diagnostic tool. Patients find it amusing to stick out their tongues but remember, your tongue is unique - it is the only organ of your body that is both interior and exterior. This is why your tongue plays an important role in TCM diagnosis. When I examine your tongue, I gain information about your body's constitution; what is going on inside you.

When I see new patients at their first appointments, and again during many of their follow-up visits, I ask them to stick out their tongues. For those of you who have not yet visited a practitioner of Chinese Medicine, the interest in your tongue may surprise you, but tongue diagnosis enables your practitioner to come to some wise conclusions about how to treat you. Just like all facets of TCM, tongue diagnosis is a very unique process; it is never one-size-fits-all.

Once you get used to the idea of your tongue as a significant element of diagnosis in Chinese Medicine, you begin to appreciate that each tongue has something to say (pun intended). In my work, I've examined puffy purple tongues, yellow coated tongues, and fire engine red tongues. Not only did Nature make tongues different from person to person, but your tongue changes as you age and as the state of your health improves or

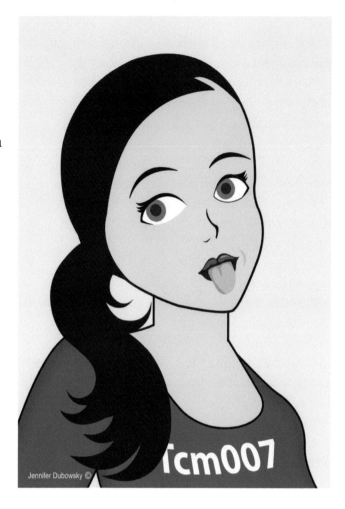

declines, providing a window into how your body is functioning.

Inspecting Your Tongue

When I examine your tongue, I do it in good light, preferably a natural light. I ask you to stick out your tongue moderately far, not too far because that can distort both its shape and color, and not too little. Tongue diagnosis is quick, easy and painless.

All tongues have imperfections so please do not become hyper-critical if you look in the mirror and check your tongue against the different criteria I describe.

What Is Your Tongue Telling Me?

I think about many aspects of your well being when I look at your tongue and, if you are interested in knowing the details, ask your practitioner to tell you what she is seeing when she checks your tongue, but for us in this chapter, I want to provide the important basics so that you can be informed about your health.

When a Chinese Medicine practitioner looks at your tongue, she observes **Shape and Size, Color,** and **Coating**. Let me tell you a little about each.

1. **Shape and Size** - The size and shape of the tongue tells me about the fluids in your body. For example, Mr. A. has a large, puffy, tongue with teeth marks that indict the fluids are not flowing through his body as freely as they should be. In contrast, a small, short tongue may indicate an insufficient amount of moisture in the body.

2. **Color** - Ideally your tongue body should have a pink and vital appearance. However, it is common to see purple and red, in varying degrees and on different parts of the tongue. Color may vary. As an example, let's continue with Mr. A., the patient above, where the shape and size of his tongue was puffy and large. Now we add information about color. If this tongue is also purplish, it indicates that the blood (one type of fluid in the body) is not flowing well throughout his body or through one part of his body. In TCM, this would be called blood stagnation. The darker the purple, the more stagnant the blood. This type of tongue might mean that Mr. A. is experiencing pain or stress or both. Red indicates heat; the redder the tongue, the greater the amount of heat. In contrast, a pale tongue could mean that there is not enough heat in the body, or that there is a deficiency of qi or blood. The tongue body rarely changes quickly. When it comes to looking at the color of your tongue, I always keep in mind that the foods you eat may have temporarily stained your tongue. I remember when a patient showed up with a very bright red tongue. Before coming to any conclusions, I asked her several questions and after a minute or two, she remembered the red lolly pop she had eaten earlier.

3. **Coating** - Coating is also called 'fur' A healthy tongue is naturally pink with a thin white coating. Unlike the tongue body, the color of the tongue coating can change quickly.

When I check the tongue coating, I look for:

    a). Thickness - Is the coating thick, thin, or nonexistent? If you are catching a cold, flu, or virus, you will see a thicker coating develop. No coating is a sign of a more severe heat or dryness. This is sometimes seen during menopause which is a time when women's bodies start to heat up; think hot flashes.

    b). Consistency - The consistency (dry or moist) of the coating is another indicator of the state of the fluids in your body. A dry coating represents a drier body just as an excessively moist coating indicates a damp body or poor fluid circulation. Lifestyle choices affect the coatings, for example, regular smokers will often have a drier, yellowish fur.

    c). Color - Just like there are different colors of the tongue, there are different colors of the fur. A thin white coating is normal. A yellow coat is a heat sign, and a gray or black coat indicates a severe condition.

    Tongue color can also vary on different parts of the tongue and I explain that next.

Your Tongue Is A Map Of Your Organs

    In Chinese medicine, the tongue provides a map of the organs. As you can see on the diagram on the next page, different parts of the tongue correlate to different organs. Liver and Gallbladder are represented by the sides of the tongue so, if the tongue is red in that particular area, it represents heat in the Liver and Gallbladder.

    Therefore, pathological changes in a certain portion of your tongue can indicate pathological changes in the corresponding organ. However, the TCM view of organs is not identical to the Western view and you might misunderstand the meaning of the changes unless you are trained in tongue diagnosis. For example, in TCM, the tip of the tongue represents the heart in an emotional sense. Practically, this means that when your tongue has a very red tip (heart in the emotional sense) it's quite likely to be your Shen (spirit/emotions) that is disturbed.

Your tongue is pretty amazing when you think about the vast amount of information it offers. I hope you now have a greater appreciation of how important your tongue is and how valuable a tool it can be in uncovering what imbalances exist, both physically and emotionally.

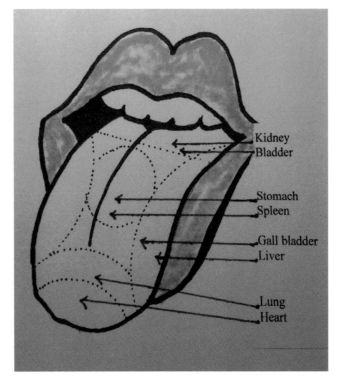

► Pulse Diagnosis

Pulse diagnosis in Traditional Chinese Medicine is unlike other forms of pulse-taking. You have certainly had the experience of sitting in your doctor's office and having your heart/pulse rate checked. If the rate, which is normally between 60-90 beats per minute, was too fast, too slow, or irregular, your physician probably spoke to you about it and may have shown some concern. It is different when you visit your practitioner of Traditional Chinese Medicine. She isn't just looking for a deviation from the 'norm' because, in TCM, your pulse reveals much more than just your heart rate. Pulse diagnosis requires subtlety and experience; it is an incredibly complex subject, and a sometimes frustrating endeavor, because it is an art as well as a science. Just as your tongue provides important information about the interior of your body, your pulses reveal information about the state of your internal organs, emotions and reflects the general health of your entire body. We feel not only for the rate but also for the **depth, length**, and **quality** of your pulses.

When I take your pulse, I place three of my fingers on three sections of the radial artery of your wrist and feel for each section of the pulse: front, middle and rear. Each section corresponds to different organs as you can see in the diagram.

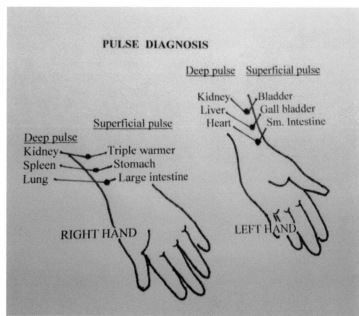

Depth, Length And Quality Of Pulses

Pulse Depth - There are also three levels of pulses: superficial, middle and deep. To feel your pulse at the most superficial level, I press very lightly. I exert a bit more pressure to read the middle, and more firmly (close to the bone) to feel the deepest level of pulse. The depth of the pulse gives me information about any pathological condition that might be present. For example: a deep pulse reflects the state of the organs and more internal conditions. However a pulse felt at the superficial level is usually a sign of an exterior illness, like a cold or flu.

Pulse Length - The length of your pulse, shorter vs. longer, provides indications of the strength and balance of blood and energy flow. Generally a longer pulse is not a concern and is often considered normal. However a shorter pulse means your energy and blood are not flowing well. Two common reasons for this are:

1. The energy is not strong enough to move your blood and this is felt as a shorter, weak pulse.

2. The blood is not flowing well because there are blockages and this is represented by a short, forceful pulse.

How can I tell if a pulse is short or long? I place three fingers on your radial artery: if the pulse is not felt under all 3 fingers, it is considered shorter; if the pulse exceeds the 3 fingers, it is considered to be longer.

Pulse Quality - Quality refers to the texture, meaning how your pulse feels under my fingers. This gives further information about the state of your health. There are 28 different pulse qualities and I will not go through all of them. As an example, two common pulse qualities are wiry and slippery. To understand a wiry pulse, imagine feeling a guitar wire or taut rope under your fingers. This type of pulse is usually felt if someone is stressed, in pain or both. I find this pulse to be quite common in my practice. Another popular pulse, especially in women, is the slippery pulse. The sensation is like of a strand of pearls running beneath my fingers. This pulse can indicate damp in the body but is common in women because of the menstrual cycle. A female has a slippery pulse when she is menstruating and when pregnant.

Putting together the different variables - depth, length, quality - of pulse diagnosis, here is a common example: a pulse might be of medium depth, fast, normal length, and wiry. A person with this type of pulse is probably pretty stressed, irritable, and maybe in pain as well. He or she would be a good candidate for acupuncture!

Not every practitioner will always feel the same thing and your pulses can change quickly so, the pulses that I feel at the beginning of your visit may differ from those I detect at the end. For example, if your pain and/or stress level has greatly diminished by the end of a session, your pulse may have slowed down a bit or feel less 'wiry'. This would be a nice outcome for a session.

Chapter 10 -What To Expect On Your First Visit

You've almost finished this book; you've heard about the many benefits of Chinese Medicine and you have decided to give TCM a try. So, what should you expect and how can you best prepare for your first appointment? Here are some basic guidelines about clothing, food, 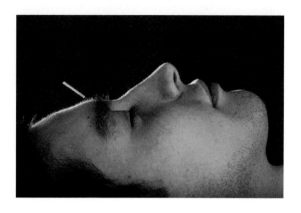 paperwork, your initial exam, and appointment frequency, although procedures may vary depending on your practitioner.

Clothing

Wear comfortable clothing so you can lie down and rest easily. For needling, you want your clothing to be loose enough so that you can roll up the legs of your pants or sleeves of your shirt. You may be offered a dressing gown, just like the Western doctors use and you can wear it or keep your own clothing on, whatever you prefer.

Food

Eat some light food before you arrive. Generally, it feels better to have acupuncture when your stomach is neither empty nor full.

Paperwork

It is a good idea to arrive a few minutes early for your first appointment because you will be asked to fill out forms about your health history. You can prepare for this by bringing along a list of your medicines, supplements, surgeries, allergies, and past treatments. The more information that your acupuncturist has about your health and your history, the better she is able to help you. Your practitioner will then ask you more questions - a good history is essential.

Initial Examination

Your practitioner will look at your tongue and take your pulse. In Chapter 9, I explained the importance of pulse and tongue diagnosis. Depending on your complaint and the information she has collected from the exam, the paperwork and your conversation, she will provide you with the appropriate treatment and other dietary or lifestyle suggestions. Treatment usually includes acupuncture treatment and herbal formulas. Your practitioner might suggest other modalities such as tui na, cupping and moxabustion. Feel free, as always, to ask what has led her to suggest these treatments and what are the goals.

Appointments And Treatment Frequency

Many people feel an improvement after just one treatment but usually additional treatments, especially in the case of longstanding problems, are required to sustain lasting results. New patients sometimes ask me, "Why do I have to come to acupuncture so often?" It is a particularly relevant question in a society like ours where most people visit doctors to 'fix' a broken part rather than using their healthcare practitioner to play an important role in keeping them healthy. Traditional Chinese Medicine has a different philosophy and a different practice. Acupuncture, Chinese herbs, and cupping are healing and do a wonderful job of repairing you, but my philosophy is not that you are broken, but that you are out of balance. In Chinese Medicine, the onset of serious or uncomfortable symptoms indicates that you've been unhealthy and out of balance prior to your uncomfortable symptom – maybe for a long time!

How Many Treatments?

The number of acupuncture treatments needed depends on you and on the length of time that your problem has existed. If your difficulty has bothered you for years, you will need a good deal more treatment than someone else who wrenched his back last week. In the latter case, maybe only a couple of treatments are needed. It will depend on the extent of your body's imbalance and how quickly your body responds. Even then, treatments are still more effective when you have them closer together, especially in the beginning. The most effective way to use acupuncture is to start with appointments that are scheduled within 2 or 3 days of each other and slow them down as you feel the good results.

The goal of Chinese Medicine is to return you to a healthy state of being, one in which your symptoms don't return. This takes time. Your body has work to do to reclaim and sustain health. Think of it as similar to taking a course of antibiotics regularly for a period of time in order to kill the infection; one strong pill is not enough to last. Acupuncture often will give you relief quickly, sometimes immediately, but to sustain the results, you need treatments over time.

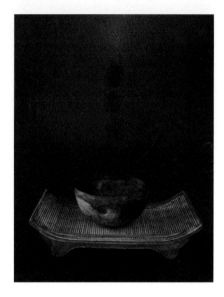

Conclusion

I love adventure! Ever since I can remember I've had a deep desire to travel and visit new places. I called my book, *Adventures in Chinese Medicine* because learning about TCM is a grand adventure! It is a chance to visit a new place and find something wonderful. Years ago, my sister and I, along with my two cats, took a long driving trip through some pretty unexciting territory. We expected some difficulties (cats don't appreciate car travel) and a little boredom but instead, we discovered a treasure in the form of a fun dome at a hotel in Lincoln, Nebraska. Other more exotic trips have provided me adventure by mesmerizing me with history and intriguing new ideas. When I walked through the streets of Rome, it became clear that this was a city that could father Caesar and rule the world. In Costa Rica, one of the most beautiful countries I've ever visited, a nighttime hike became an encounter with armies of marching ants. I learned to take the guides seriously when they suggest wearing long pants tucked into my socks for night treks in the forest, forget fashion!

Many of my adventures have come from travel, but some of the best were provided by studying Chinese Medicine. My experiences in Asia were amazing. China is a beautiful and ancient country. I got to spend time at a hospital in Beijing and it really fortified my love of Chinese Medicine. I witnessed firsthand how all forms of Traditional Chinese Medicine were incorporated into their health system, and I saw the effectiveness of using acupuncture, cupping, herbs and tui na in a hospital setting, something that is still rare here.

My work in Traditional Chinese Medicine has provided me with different ways to think about our relationship with the world around us, phenomenal ways of healing, and endless opportunities. When I invited you into *Adventures in Chinese Medicine,* I hoped that you would feel my passion and develop a little of your own. I sincerely hope that your journey with Chinese Medicine's ideas and practices is just beginning, not ending, go further and step from reading about these ideas into experiencing acupuncture, herbal remedies and more. It has been my joy to be your guide.

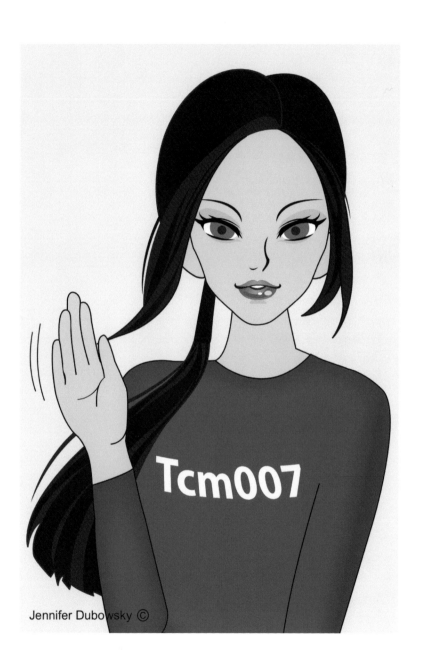

Jennifer Dubowsky ©

Resources

Jennifer Dubowsky, L.A.c.
325 W. Huron Street, suite # 308
Chicago, Illinois 60654
Phone: 312-399-5098
tcm007.com
acupuncturechicago.blogspot.com

Linda Edelstein, P.h.D.
636 Church Street, suite # 422
Evanston, Illinois 60201
Phone: 847-328-7878
therapyevanston.com

Diane M. Lowry, L.A.c.
HealthFocus Acupuncture and Oriental Medicine
5030 Sadler Place, suite # 202
Glen Allen, Virginia 23060
Phone: 804-467-1355
HealthFocusAcupuncture.com

Nicole Hohmann, L.A.c.
2400 Chestnut Ave, Suite A
Glenview, Illinois 60026
Phone: 847-657-3540
nicolehohmann@yahoo.com

Kai Tao, ND, MPH, CNM
ktao@post.harvard.edu

Azhar Ehasn
Art Director/CEO
Ha-meem Multimedia
0092 322 6919921

Here are some helpful websites with articles about Chinese Medicine and/or resources to find a qualified acupuncturist near you.

N.C.C.A.O.M. - National Certification Commission for Acupuncture and Oriental Medicine nccaom.org
acufinder.com
acupuncturetoday.com

Selected Research Studies

Topic: Acupuncture Improves Fertility

Influence of acupuncture on the pregnancy rate in patients who undergo assisted reproduction therap.y Wolfgang E. Paulus, M.D., Mingmin Zhang, M.D., Erwin Strehler, M.D., Imam El Danasouri, Ph.D., and Karl Sterzik, M.D. Fertility and Sterility. Vol. 77, # 4, April, 2002.

Results - A German study followed 160 women, providing acupuncture to 80 subjects with their IVF treatments. The results were significant: "The analysis shows that the pregnancy rate for the acupuncture group is considerably higher than for the control group (42.5% vs. 26.3%)."

Effects of acupuncture on pregnancy rates in women undergoing in vitro fertilization: a systematic review and meta-analysis. Cui Hong Zheng, M.D., Ph.D.a, Guang Ying Huang, M.D., Ph.D.a, Ming Min Zhang, M.D., Ph.D.b, Wei Wang, M.D., Ph.D.c.. Fertility and Sterility. January, 2012.

Results - Acupuncture improved pregnancy and live birth rates.

Effects of acupuncture on rates of pregnancy and live birth among women undergoing in vitro fertilization: systematic review and meta-analysis. E. Manheimer, G. Zhang, L. Udoff et al. British Medical Journal. February, 2008; 336:545-549. PubMed.

Results - Acupuncture increased the chances of pregnancy during IVF treatments by 65%.

Acupuncture on the day of embryo transfer significantly improves the reproductive outcome in infertile women: a prospective, randomized trial. L.G. Westergaard, Q. Mao, M. Krogslund, S. Sandrini, S. Lenz, and J. Grinsted. Fertility and Sterility. April, 2006:1341-1346.

Results - Acupuncture administered on the day of embryo transfer significantly improved the reproductive outcome of IVF or ICSI as compared with no acupuncture.

Changes in serum cortisol and prolactin associated with acupuncture during IVF. P.C. Magarelli, D. Cridennda, M. Cohen. Fertility and Sterility, December, 2009; 92(6):1870-9.

Results - The pregnancy and live birth rate was significantly higher in the acupuncture group. The women in the acupuncture group also showed beneficial changes in their levels of stress hormones. The acupuncture seemed to help normalize the cortisol and prolactin levels of the women as compared to the control group who did not have acupuncture. This could improve both egg quality and implantation.

Quantitative evaluation of spermatozoa ultrastructure after acupuncture treatment for idiopathic male infertility J.Pei, Ph.D., E. Strehler, M.D., U. Noss, M.D., M.Abt, Ph.D., P. Piomboni, Ph.D., B. Baccetti, Ph.D., K. Sterzik, M.D. Fertility and Sterility July, 2005, 84(1): 141-147.

Results - Acupuncture helped infertile men by improving sperm quality in their semen.

Impact of electro-acupuncture and physical exercise on hyperandrogenism and oligo/amenorrhea in women with polycystic ovary syndrome: a randomized controlled trial. Elizabeth Jedel, Fernand Labrie, Anders Odén, Göran Holm, Lars Nilsson, Per Olof Janson, Anna-Karin Lind, Claes Ohlsson, and Elisabet Stener-Victorin. American J Physiology, Endocrinology, Metabolism 2011, 300: E37–E45.

Results - Electro-acupuncture improved menstrual frequency and balanced sex steroid levels in women with polycystic ovarian syndrome (PCOS).

Topic: Pain Relief

Adenosine A1 receptors mediate local anti-nociceptive effects of acupuncture. N. Goldman, M. Chen, T. Fujita, Q. Xu, W. Peng, W. Liu, TK. Jensen, Y. Pei, F. Wang, X. Han, JF. Chen, J. Schnermann, T. Takano, L. Bekar, K.A. Tieu, M. Nedergaard. Nature Neuroscience published online May 30th, 2010.

Results - This study links acupuncture to the stimulation of a chemical compound called adenosine in the body. Adenosine is a painkiller naturally manufactured when the body is injured.

Traditional Chinese acupuncture and placebo (sham) acupuncture are differentiated by their effects on-opioid receptors (MORs). Richard E. Harris, Jon-Kar Zubieta, David J. Scott, Vitaly Napadow, Richard H. Gracely, Daniel J. Clauw. Journal of NeuroImage, V. 47(3): 1077-1085, September 2009.

74

Results - Using brain imaging, researchers at the U-M Chronic Pain and Fatigue Research Center were the first to provide evidence that traditional Chinese acupuncture affects the brain's long-term ability to regulate pain. Acupuncture increased the binding availability of mu-opoid receptors in regions of the brain that process and dampen pain signals. Opioid painkillers, include drugs like morphine and codeine which are thought to work by binding to these opioid receptors in the brain and spinal cord.

Acupuncture for tension-type headache. K. Linde et al. Cochrane Database of Systematic Reviews, Issue 1. Art. No.: CD007587 DOI: 10.1002/14651858.CD007587
Acupuncture for migraine prophylaxis. K. Linde et al. Cochrane Database of Systematic Reviews, 2009, Issue 1. Art.No.: CD001218 DOI 10.1002/14651858.CD001218.pub2

Results - Two separate systematic reviews by Cochrane Researchers showed that acupuncture is an effective treatment for prevention of headaches and migraines.

A combined [11C]diprenorphine PET study and fMRI study of acupuncture analgesia. M. Webb, D. Dougherty, J. Kong, A. Bonab, A. Fischman, and R. Gollub. Behavioural Brain Research, V193(1): 63-68, November, 2008.

Results - The study explains how acupuncture reduces pain. Harvard scientists used a PET Scan (Positron emission tomography) with functional magnetic resonance imaging (fMRI) to examine brain signals and pain receptors during an acupuncture analgesia treatment. Both showed changes in several portions of the brain. Researchers concluded that acupuncture changes the already existing brain opioids which are central to the experience of pain.

Topic: Acupuncture Increases Blood Flow to the Brain

Effects of GV20 Acupuncture on Cerebral Blood Flow Velocity of Middle Cerebral Artery and Anterior Cerebral Artery Territories, and CO2 Reactivity During Hypocapnia in Normal Subjects. Hyung-sik Byeon, Sang-kwan Moon, Seong-uk Park, Woo-sang Jung, Jung-mi Park, Chang-nam Ko, Ki-ho Cho, Young-suk Kim and Hyung-sup Bae. The Journal of Alternative and Complementary Medicine. 17(3): 219-224, March, 2011.

Results - Research showed that acupuncture at acupoint GV20 also known as DU20, (located on the top of the head) increases blow flow to the brain without raising blood pressure or pulse rate.

Topic: Acupuncture Reduced Hot Flashes

Menopausal Symptom Management With Acupuncture For Women With Breast Cancer. S. Cohen, M. Rousseau, J. Berg, R. Jolivet , L. Dixon , J. Vulte, J. Kern. WebmedCentral ALTERNATIVE MEDICINE 2011;2(2):WMC001544.

Results - A Yale University/University of Pittsburg study of women with hot flashes brought on by conventional breast cancer treatment reveals that women who received acupuncture had a 30% reduction in hot flashes.

Bio

Jennifer Dubowsky is a licensed acupuncturist with a practice in downtown Chicago, Illinois, since 2002. Jennifer earned her Bachelor of Science degree in Kinesiology from University of Illinois in Chicago and her Master of Science degree in Oriental Medicine from Southwest Acupuncture College, an accredited 4 year Masters program in Boulder, Colorado. She received her Diplomate from the NCCAOM, the National Certification Commission for Acupuncture and Oriental Medicine and completed an internship at the Sino-Japanese Friendship Hospital in Beijing, China. Jennifer has a passion for her work and has researched and written articles on Chinese medicine, given talks, created a seasonal newsletter and maintains a popular blog about health and Chinese Medicine, Acupuncture Blog Chicago (acupuncturechicago.blogspot.com). Adventures in Chinese Medicine is her first book.

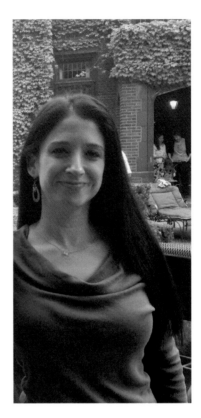

CPSIA information can be obtained
at www.ICGtesting.com
Printed in the USA
LVIC07n0212100713
342178LV00006B